The Cancer Prevention Handbook

Steve Riczo

The Cancer Prevention Handbook

Contents

Acknowledgements (listed alphabetically)

The author would like to gratefully acknowledge the following universities, cancer centers, medical schools, and other organizations such as the National Institute of Environmental Health Science for making one or more of their experts available to be interviewed by the author in order to advance peoples knowledge about cancer prevention.

Albert Einstein College of Medicine

Barnes-Jewish Hospital, St. Louis Siteman Cancer Center

Brown University

Boise State University

California State University

Clemson University

Cleveland Clinic Taussig Cancer Institute

Colorado State University

Cornell University Center for Behavior Economics

Dartmouth College Dartmouth Medical School

Dayton Clinical Oncology Group

East Carolina University Brady School of Medicine Leo W. Jenkins Cancer Center

Eastern Michigan University

Eastern Virginia Medical School

Florida State University

Francis Marion University

Georgetown University

Harvard University

Indiana State University

Indiana University of
Pennsylvania

Kent State University

Louisiana State University
Stanly S. Scott Cancer Center

Metagenics

Moffitt Cancer Center

Medical University of South
Carolina
Hollings Cancer Center

Northern Arizona University

National Institute of
Environmental Health Science
(NIH)

Northeastern State University

Northern Kentucky University

Ohio State University
James Comprehensive Cancer
Center

Old Dominion University

Oklahoma State University

Oklahoma Tobacco Research
Center

Penn State Hershey Cancer
Institute

Portland State University

Plymouth State University

Princeton University

Sanford Burnham Laboratory

Stanford University
Stanford Cancer Institute

State University of New York at
Geneseo

Thomas Jefferson University
Kimmel Cancer Center

Tufts University School of
Medicine

UMass School of Public Health
Sciences

University of Arizona Cancer
Center

University of California
Berkeley
School of Public Health

University of California, Davis

University of California, San
Diego
Moores Comprehensive Cancer
Center

University of California, San
Diego
Center for Integrative
Medicine

University of California, San
Francisco
Helen Diller Family
Comprehensive Cancer Center

University of California, Santa
Barbara

University of Colorado Cancer
Center

University of Florida

University of Georgia

University of Hawaii Cancer
Center

University of Houston

University of Illinois

University of Iowa
Holden Comprehensive Cancer
Center

University of Kansas Medical
Center

University of Kentucky
Markey Cancer Center

University of Kentucky College
of Medicine

University of Louisiana

University of Louisville

University of Memphis School
of Public Health

University of Minnesota

University of Missouri School of
Medicine
Ellis Fischel Cancer Center

University of North Carolina, Chapel Hill

University of North Florida

University of Oklahoma Health Sciences Center
Stephenson Cancer Center

University of Pittsburgh

University of Texas Health Science Center
Memorial Hermann Cancer Center

University of Tennessee Cancer Institute

University of Utah
Huntsman Cancer Institute

Utah State University

Virginia Commonwealth University
Massey Cancer Center

Yale University School of Medicine
Yale Cancer Center

Wake Forest Baptist Medical Center

Washington State University

Wayne State University
Barbara Ann Karmanos Cancer Institute

Wichita State University

Dedication

This book is dedicated to my son Dan, my daughter Sarah, Sarah's dear friend Kelly who was diagnosed with cancer, all of the cancer patients who courageously fight this terrible disease and to all of their physicians who fight it with them as well as to cancer researchers and cancer epidemiologists throughout the world who dedicate their lives to trying to find cures and the best ways to prevent cancer from occurring in the first place.

Section I

Introduction, Causes of Cancer and

Case for Prevention

1

Introduction

This year, over 580,000 Americans will die from what experts believe to be a largely preventable disease - cancer. To put that number in perspective, that is more than all the US servicemen and women who died in action during the wars in Afghanistan, Iraq, Vietnam, Korea and World War II - combined. It is the number one killer in the United States for people under the age of 85. Cancer is not just something that happens to other people – almost all Americans have someone in their lives who have had cancer. The lifetime risk of getting cancer is one out of three for women and one out of two for men. In other words, if you know nine women or girls, statistically three of them will get cancer at some point during their lives. If you know 10 boys or men, five of them will get cancer. The World Health Organization predicts significant increases in cancer worldwide.

Why is it that more than 40 years after the President of the United States declared a War on Cancer with the signing of the National Cancer Act of 1971 that set a goal of finding a cure for cancer that we still cannot declare victory and a cure is nowhere in sight? What can individuals and families do to prevent this dreaded disease, or for those who already have been diagnosed with cancer, prevent it from metastasizing (spreading within the body) and living a lifestyle that prolongs their lives? Can we someday win the war on cancer, and if so, how do we need to adjust current strategies in that war?

What is cancer? Cancer is a term used for diseases in which an abnormal cell divides without control which are then able to invade other tissues and organs via the blood and lymph systems which is called metastasis. Metastatic cancer is cancer that has spread from the place where it first started to another place in the body. According to the National Cancer Institute, cancer starts with mutations in the genes within a cell that cause it to change from a normal cell to a cancer cell. Steven McMahon, Ph.D., Professor of Epigenetics at Thomas Jefferson University says, "Most cancers arise through a single mutation in one of our 20,000 genes...". While all cancers involve gene mutations, the vast majority of cancers are not inevitably determined by inherited defective genes from our parents but rather triggered through an interaction of our genes and environment. A gene mutation, regardless of the cause, if not resolved by our immune system, can adversely affect the cell in which it resides.

Erin Eaton, Ph.D., Associate Professor of Biology at Francis Marion University notes, "All cancers start from a single cell." Christine Curran, Ph.D., Assistant Professor of Biology at Northern Kentucky University adds, "Cancer is unregulated cell growth. They divide and divide and they are not supposed to do that." While many people think of cancer as being organ specific such as lung cancer (which causes the most cancer deaths in both men and women), skin, breast, prostate, cervical, pancreas, brain, kidney and colon, experts say that it is actually many diseases characterized by a variety of genetic mutations that take place within our cells. Dean Hosgood, Ph.D., M.P.H., at Albert Einstein College of Medicine notes:

> Cancers are a multitude of diseases, hundreds if not thousands of different diseases... We traditionally thought of them sort of organ specific...but now in the molecular age, we are able to more accurately divide these cancers into subtypes based on their molecular characteristics and how they are acting in the body.

Anthony Shield, M.D., Associate Director of the Barbara Ann Karmanos Cancer Institute at Wayne State University concurs adding, "Cancer is not just one disease but probably 100 or 1000 diseases."

In the United States, some cancers are declining but others are increasing unexplainably including childhood cancers. Robert Hiatt M.D., Ph.D., Chair, Department of Epidemiology at the University of California, San Francisco notes, "For thyroid cancer, that could be environmental chemicals but I don't think we have a clue. For brain cancer, we don't have a clue". Cancer is so prevalent that it is a major concern to people. Many who experience one or more physical symptoms worry that it might be cancer. Jeff Bland, Ph.D., President of the Personalized Lifestyle Medicine Institute says, "I think if you really ask people their deeper thoughts, I think you'll find virtually every adult is worried about cancer and it is at the back of their mind." It is a dreaded disease that happens to real people and their families and loved ones whose lives are never the same again once they hear these words from their physician, "You have cancer". It is at that mind-numbing moment that the patient realizes his or her life will never be the same again. Paul Walker, M.D., Clinical Associate Professor and Director of Oncology at the Brady School of Medicine at East Carolina University notes, "After the cancer diagnosis, everybody, rightly or wrongly, when realizing 'I have cancer', the first thing they think of is, 'I am going to die' – that's what hits you in the face and the gut."

Why is there so much pessimism about the cancer diagnosis? Mainly, because a true permanent "cure" for most cancer patients does not really exist. According to the National Cancer Institute (NCI), "A cure means that treatment has eradicated all traces of a person's cancer...but does not mean that the person will never have cancer again. It is possible that another cancer, even the same type of cancer, will develop in the person's body at some point in the future." In addition, most American adults have seen a family member, friend, neighbor or coworker struggle with cancer including the debilitating side effects of current cancer treatments especially chemotherapy that often include hair loss and nausea or worse or have lost someone near and dear to them to the disease. Luoping Zhang, Ph.D., a toxicologist and Professor of Environmental Health Sciences at the University of California, Berkeley School of Public Health says, "Cancer patients who are treated for their primary cancer with chemotherapeutic drugs which are highly toxic can cause secondary cancer in the form of leukemia that is a result of the treatment." Aliasger Salem, Ph.D., Professor of Pharmaceutical Science at the University of Iowa and Holden Comprehensive Cancer Center explains, "...chemotherapy has an adverse effect on cancer cells but also an adverse effect on healthy cells so patients suffer these very, very serious side effects as part of the therapy such as hair loss, nausea, weakness, those types of things and they are pretty significant." Too many cancer patients receive chemotherapy in clinical trials (experimental) who receive no benefit and may actually be worse off as it often makes their final days or months miserable by suffering terrible side effects from the highly toxic chemotherapy drugs.

One document from an NCI accredited cancer center stated that 90% of the patients who receive chemotherapy in clinical trials (experimental) do not benefit from the treatment which should not to be confused with patients receiving chemotherapy that is no longer experimental and is in widespread use. The current philosophy being taught by many clinicians is to simply treat a big group of cancer patients with chemotherapy in clinical trials and some will likely benefit. The problem is that harm can also be done to many of them and patients often do not fully understand the risks. East Carolina University's Dr. Walker explains:

> Let's say it [chemotherapy in a clinical trial] does not work in 90% [of patients], what about the 10% that it does?... That median survival that we all talk about [for lung cancer

patients] is that 50th person out of 100 and has nothing to do with the other 99. NCI talks about changing the clinical trial process but really have not stepped it up to where I think it needs to be...Everybody says we have to treat 100 to benefit four [cancer patients]. Well, if you apply it that way, yes, but NCI Canada did a gene expression profile on their patients that had stage IB and 2 lung cancers and they were able to identify the two thirds that were going to do great without chemotherapy, and the one third that were going to die no matter what – if they didn't get chemotherapy. Then when they looked at the study, of those who were going to die, 70% were cured by adding the chemotherapy. Conversely, those that were going to do great, 20% died, there was a lower survival, because you are doing harm when a person does not need it. The problem is there is no readily commercially available way to know who really needs what...Progress is being made but it still very, very, very frustratingly slow...I teach the hematology-oncology fellows we learn from groups but we take care of individuals. The mindset in the guidelines is we just take care of the group and we don't have to individualize anything. You can do incredible benefit...but are also doing harm.

Dr. Walker added that patients often do not fully understand the nuances and risks of the actual harm that can be caused by the chemotherapeutic drug and patients generally simply trust their oncologist to 'tell me what you think is best'.

This is not to say that that there has not been any progress in the War on Cancer. Although we are not yet winning the war, we have won some important battles which deservedly should be recognized and celebrated as researchers in the United States and throughout the world are working hard every day to try to come up with solutions. In spite of the large absolute numbers of cancer deaths, mortality rates from cancer in the US are going down by about 1% per year which means patients with cancer are living longer. Furthermore, techniques have been developed to detect some cancers early which are often very treatable which offers substantial improvement in the prognosis for those patients – they can often live much longer than they would have otherwise. John Vena, Ph.D., Professor of Epidemiology at the Medical University of South Carolina explains, "Early diagnosis and prompt treatment of cancer is really important…". East Carolina's Dr. Paul Walker adds, "Medical oncologists get excited about new advances but what it really comes down to, by golly, is with early detection, who needs new advances." Well-known examples of early cancer detection methods include mammography for breast cancer, colonoscopy for colon cancer, PSA for prostate cancer and PAP tests for cervical cancer.

With some cancers, such as breast cancer, improvements in early detection and treatment help patients to live considerably longer than would have otherwise been the case. Nicole Simone, M.D., Radiation Oncologist at Thomas Jefferson University points out that, "Breast cancer nowadays is very curable - we actually look at it like almost a chronic disease." Dean Hosgood, Ph.D., M.P.H., at Albert Einstein College of Medicine concurs adding that with "early detection of breast cancer now, many people with breast cancer are surviving 10, 20, 30, 40, even 50 years…". Today in America, there are about 13 million cancer survivors which is defined as anyone who has been diagnosed with cancer and is still living. Many of them have benefited from early cancer detection techniques. For many whose cancer is diagnosed very early and is localized (has not metastasized or spread), this is as close to a "cure" as is possible since there is a higher risk for reoccurrence in individuals who have been diagnosed with cancer than for those who have not. Thomas Kensler, Ph.D., Professor of Cancer Pharmacology and Cancer Prevention at the University of Pittsburgh says, "If everybody in this country was getting screened for colorectal cancer according to current screening guidelines, then the estimate is that probably at least one third of colorectal cancers would be prevented." John Kellogg Parsons, M.D., Associate Professor at the University of California, San Diego Moores Comprehensive Cancer Center adds, "Prostate cancer is the number one diagnosed cancer among men and the second leading cause of cancer death in the United States...men should be tested with the PSA test beginning around the age of 45 to 50."

There are also some emerging developments in cancer treatment, including targeted chemotherapy and immunotherapy, using chemotherapeutic agents and the body's own immune system respectively to attack cancer cells directly while attempting to minimize toxicity to surrounding tissues and organs which is a common problem with today's standard chemotherapy. However, experts note that there are many technical hurdles ahead with these new technologies and only time will tell whether they will prove to be helpful for most cancer patients. Currently, the standard treatments for most cancers are surgery, chemotherapy and radiation therapy which, in spite of the aforementioned progress, all have their limitations in terms of totally eradicating the cancer from patients. Jeff Bland, Ph.D., President of the Personalized Lifestyle Medicine Institute explains, "We know the facts about cancer treatment. They are still not good." Richard Heller, Ph.D., Professor of Medical Laboratory and Radiation Sciences at Old Dominion University says while chemotherapy can have a positive impact in some cases, "Many times, chemotherapy does not have that big of a success rate...". According to the National Cancer Institute, "Although some types of metastatic cancer can be cured with current treatments, most cannot." Why has it been so difficult to develop effective treatments and come up with a cure for cancer? In addition to the many types of cancers noted above, cancer cells can be remarkably persistent and resilient. Howard Gross, M.D., a medical oncologist with the Dayton Clinical Oncology Program says, "Cancer cells are sometimes smarter than we are. They get knocked down and then they sneak around and come up with a resistance mechanism that fools us all."

Some people like to point out that although we have a high incidence of cancer, people generally live longer today than they did in the past. While it is true that some people live longer, unfortunately, cancer patients are often not able to live to the average life expectancy to enjoy the longevity of life enjoyed by so many others who do not get cancer. In fact, actuarial data suggests that cancer patients lose 15 years of their life on average. In addition, a significant part of the statistical difference in our longer lifespan today vs. the distant past can be attributed to a higher infant and childhood mortality rate in the past. Michael Gurven, Ph.D., an Evolutionary Anthropologist from the University of California, Santa Barbara, who is well-versed in Evolutionary Medicine, explains:

> Even though life expectancies are much smaller in hunter gatherer types of populations, what it usually means is that those are averages over the life course with infant mortality being very high - up to 200 times higher in hunter gatherer societies that in the modern US...If one survived to age 15, then it's not as dramatically different as you would think as there's a good chance that you could make it until age 60...

There are far too many cancer patients today who, even in this world of 21st century modern medicine, do not live to age 60.

2

Causes of Cancer

What causes cancer? Many cancers are thought to result from multiple contributing factors. Ann Schwartz, Ph.D., Deputy Center Director at the Barbara Ann Karmanos Cancer Institute at Wayne State University says, "Most cancers are not caused by one thing." Contributing factors to cancer development include: cancer causing substances (carcinogens) that we get through our environment such air or water pollution or as a result of lifestyle decisions such as smoking. Other contributing factors can include a weak immune system, inherited genes, infections, hormone imbalance and aging.

Sometimes cancer is referred to as a disease of aging since, like many chronic illnesses, cancer incidence or frequency increases with age. Edward Trapido, Ph.D., Chair for Cancer Epidemiology at the Louisiana State University School of Public Health notes, "At a certain point, as people grow older...some of those mutations won't be handled by the body and they will continue to multiply and eventually become cancer...". Matthew Gage, Ph.D., Professor of Chemistry and Biochemistry at Northern Arizona University says, "Cancers come from an accumulation of mutations in the genome so the longer you live, the more exposures you are going to have...". The risk of saying that cancer is a disease of aging is that it might lead some to become complacent or even fatalistic, incorrectly believing that they cannot prevent cancer because they are getting older so why bother to prevent exposures to potential or known carcinogens. This is just the opposite of what most cancer experts believe – that many cancers are prevent-able. David Wheeler, Ph.D., Assistant Professor of Biostatistics at Virginia Commonwealth University's Massey Cancer Center says, "I would say that that probably over generalizes the association between aging and cancer. Generally, the incidence rate of cancer does increase with older people but you have childhood leukemias on the rise, for example...and you also have people who live to a very old age who do not die of cancer. It's a little bit too simplistic of a thought."

As both genetics and environment play a role in the develop-ment of most cancers, it is important that people be aware of any family history of cancer that can increase cancer risk. Peter Lance, M.D., Professor of Medicine and Chief Cancer Prevention and Control Officer at the University of Arizona explains:

> It is very important that every individual knows the kind of history of cancer there is in their own particular family. For instance, if in every generation there was a woman in the family with breast cancer or if there have been a number of people in the family with colon cancer at an early age, then that may trigger a very different and more intense approach [to lifestyle and early detection procedures] than the average...

Some people are more susceptible to getting cancer from cer-tain environmental exposures than others due to individual variabil-ity. Yawei Zhang, M.D., Ph.D. M.P.H., Associate Professor of Cancer Epidemiology at the Yale School of Medicine says, "Some people have a genetic susceptibility to cancer. Two people can have the same exposures and one person can get the disease and the other does not." Louisiana State University's Edward Trapido, Ph.D. notes, "Not everybody who smokes is going to develop cancer so there is a genetic component." Melissa Davis, Ph.D., Assistant Professor of Genetics at the University of Georgia adds:

Be very vigilant about your family history because some people are more susceptible to getting cancer than others and the clue to that is if you have a family history, whether someone in your family has ever been diagnosed with cancer before - that's the first red flag and that's one of the most important things a clinician will look at in terms of your cancer risk...A negative family history does not give you a clean bill of health...You may have cancer family history that you don't know about because it wasn't diagnosed as such...The number of people in your family who have had a certain type of cancer is also relevant and the age at which they got cancer.

Susan Arnold, M.D., Associate Professor of Medical Oncology and Radiation Medicine at the Markey Cancer Center at the University of Kentucky notes, "Family history, how you live, where you live, and your genetic makeup are all going to make a difference in the risk that you have for cancer." Kathy Baumgartner, Ph.D., Professor of Epidemiology at the University of Louisville says, "Just because you have a family history doesn't mean something bad is going to happen....[and conversely] not having a family history of breast cancer is certainly a very good thing but it is not the magic bullet that will protect you."

Alice Whittemore, Ph.D., Professor of Health Policy, Epidemiology and Biostatistics at Stanford University points out that:

Having a family history of cancer is a smoking gun that there may be genetic factors running through the family...because of the big element of chance involved, like a woman with no risk factors at all can suddenly develop breast cancer and the woman with many risk factors avoids it. It points to how little we understand about the human body and the breakthroughs we have to make with our understanding. Will we get there and 25 years? I'm not sure.

Ze'ev Ronai, Ph.D., Scientific Director of Sanford Burnham Laboratory points out that, "Some of us are genetically made up to be more susceptible than others to certain types of cancer." LSU's Dr. Trapido, Ph.D. says, "Cancer is caused by a combination of some genetic predisposition, genetic changes and the environmental exposures, and in this case, I am talking about environment with what we call a big 'E' that includes diet and tobacco and anything non-genetic."

That brings up a very important point. In spite of the role of genetics and hereditary factors, there is widespread agreement among cancer experts that most cancers are caused by an interaction between our genetics and environment. Only about 5% to 10% of all cancers are solely a result of hereditary genetic factors such as those caused by the BRCA genes in breast cancer. In other words, the vast majority of cancers are not caused solely by genes inherited from your parents. Xiaohui Xu, M.D., Ph.D., M.P.H., Professor of Environmental Epidemiology at the University of Florida's College of Public Health explains, "...the vast majority of cancers are due to an interaction between genetics and environment."

As mentioned above, while it is true that people with a family history of cancer are at increased risk, this does not mean that they will get cancer. Carlos Crespo, Ph.D., Professor of Community Health at Portland State University explains:

> There is an old saying that genetics loads the gun and environment pulls the trigger...There is not a lot we can do about our genetic makeup so some people say, 'I can't help it, I have that gene so I am going to be overweight'. But from an environmental perspective, we have control...

Gordon Saxe, M.D., Ph.D., Director for the Center for Integrative Medicine at University of California, San Diego concludes, "Ultimately, there may be some limits imposed by our genes but I think we tremendously overestimate those and we disempower ourselves in the process and it's false. It is leading us to underappreciate how much we can help ourselves." Charlie Wei, Ph.D., Professor of Cellular and Molecular Biology and Immunology at Clemson University adds, "...genetics and environment are both important." Abby Benninghoff, Ph.D., Assistant Professor of Epigenetics at Utah State University says:

> Our genes are not necessarily our destiny...There has been a growing consensus in the past 10 or15 years that we have not paid enough attention to the nurture [environment and lifestyle] side...Therefore, if we can find what those causative factors are, and remove those from our lifestyle, or identify other environmental influences like a healthy diet... then that's a strategy for trying to improve our health.

Jia-Sheng Wang, M.D., Ph.D., Professor and Head of Environmental Health Sciences at the University of Georgia adds, "Most experts in the field agree that the vast majority of cancers are caused primarily by environmental and lifestyle factors...the food we eat, the air we breathe, the water we drink...". University of Florida's Dr. Xu suggests, "Cancers have different causes and the vast majority are due to an interaction between genetics and environment. Environment plays a significant role." John Bell, M.D., Director of the Cancer Institute at the University of Tennessee says, "Control the controllable. Do the things that you can personally do by making healthy lifestyle choices that maximize your chance of both prolonging your life as well as prolonging your quality of your life...".

Evolution & Rapid Environmental Changes

While there are obvious benefits to the modern world in which we live and cancers have been found in some human remains several thousands of years old, the way we live today is totally different than the way humans evolved and is contributing to cancer development. Human evolution occurred over a very long period of time while changes in the environment and lifestyles of humans are occurring at a lightning fast speed. Robert Hiatt M.D., Ph.D., Chair, Department of Epidemiology at the University of California, San Francisco notes, "Genetic change takes place over tens of thousands of years in an evolutionary sense...". It is very likely that our bodies cannot adjust to these changes fast enough and cancer is one of the unfortunate outcomes. University of Kentucky's Susan Arnold, M.D. says, "It makes sense to me that our society has changed so much in terms of evolutionary stress and environmental toxins that we will probably not catch up."

The University of California, Santa Barbara's Michael Gurven, Ph.D. explains, "[Regarding environmental exposures] there are tons of exposures we would have not had in the past...Anything that has changed dramatically in the past, let's say, 50 years, certainly our ability to adapt genetically is 'zero'...". Since many of today's environmental toxins and other carcinogens such as cigarettes, synthetic (manmade) chemicals and industrial pollutants did not exist for most of human history, early human cancers had other causes. Rashmi Kaul, Ph.D., Associate Professor of Immunology at Oklahoma State University Center for Health Sciences explains, "What we know right now is that about 20% of all cancers are due to infectious diseases which are likely causes for some of the cancers found in remains thousands of years ago."

In order to understand cancer and the environment more clearly, it is useful to very briefly review human evolution and the environment in which our ancestors lived compared to today. Humans and our earlier ancestors have been evolving for millions of years. The first of the homo species, homo-habilis, is thought to have arrived on the scene about 2.5 million years ago. Yale University's Yong Zhu, Ph.D. notes, "Our bodies evolved for millions of years until now...". Our own species, homo-sapiens is estimated to have been around for approximately 150,000 years or so. Homo-sapiens, for the vast majority of our existence, and all of our earlier homo species were hunter gatherers who lived a completely different lifestyle in a completely different environment than we do today. They spent most of their waking time moving around from place to place foraging for food. When they used up the food supply in one place, they simply moved on to another. Unlike today, food was scarce and they burned energy through a physically demanding lifestyle. Humans also evolved with a propensity to store fat for times of extreme food scarcity or famine – a trait that does not serve us well for the most part now with our abundance of calorie dense food which contributes to obesity – a known cancer risk. Maura Harrigan, M.S., a registered dietician who is board certified in oncology nutrition with the Yale Cancer Center explains:

> There is a mismatch between how our bodies are designed to live - in an environment that requires physical activity and where food is scarce. So now we are living in this environment that we created where very little physical activity is required with this abundant food supply which tends to be high-fat, high sugar and high salt.

A major change for humans occurred with the advent of farming which began about 12,000 years ago, initially in the Middle East, and then later spread around the globe. For the first time, farming allowed people to stay in one place and as food production increased, specialization occurred – some people continued to farm while some made clothing or provided other needed goods or services in the earliest communities and villages. Many people became subsistence farmers which was still physically demanding and early economies did not allow for disposable income for most people so high caloric food, overeating and obesity were not a major problem. For almost the entire 150,000 year time period for homo sapiens, there was no burning of fossil fuels for cars, trucks, steam ships, coal burning for electricity, or factories causing air or water pollution nor were people exposed to thousands of synthetic chemicals – none of these had been invented. Then suddenly, all of that changed. Starting in the mid-1700s with the invention of the steam engine came the beginning of the industrial revolution in Europe that later spread to the United States and other countries. From all sources, pollution has become so bad that the vast majority of the world climate scientists are seriously concerned about global warming and air and water pollution. Then, starting about 70 years ago, the industrial chemical revolution began leading to the development of tens of thousands of synthetic environmental chemicals, mostly in recent decades and usually with unknown health risks, that had not existed throughout the millions of years of human evolution. Nancy Schoenberg, Ph.D., a medical anthropologist with the University of Kentucky College of Medicine notes:

> The human body has not changed significantly in thousands of years so I don't think that we adapt to the infusion of chemicals in a generation or two and from an evolutionary perspective, I think that these chemicals can wreak a lot of damage that our bodies are simply not prepared to adapt to in such a short period of time if ever at all.

Even childbirth patterns changed including having children later in life and fewer of them that experts say increases cancer risk. Dr. Gurven explains:

> The average in some hunter gatherer societies is six children and some have an average of eight children...The risk of breast cancer is 100 times higher in a modern population like the US that has this type of reproductive behavior and hormonal exposure...Modern women are at much higher risks of certain types of reproductive cancers...

The World Health Organization adds, "The causes of breast and cervical cancer are related, at least in part, to a woman's sexual and reproductive choices…age at first pregnancy and number of preg-nancies, breast-feeding history, diet and physical activity."

Why is all of this important? Simply put, the evolutionary processes that shaped our human existence occurred slowly. Throughout evolution, our bodies and immune system evolved to help protect us from many, although certainly not all, of the environmental threats that were present during most of human evolution - such as fighting off many diseases. For most of the human existence, the air was clean, the water was clean, food was relatively scarce and humans moved around a lot out of necessity to survive and their physically active lifestyle contributed to good health – there was no sedentary lifestyle if one wanted to survive. We now live in a world which is characterized by an environment and lifestyle that promote cancer risks such as: sedentary life-styles – there were no office jobs for hunter-gatherers; over-eating with commensurate obesity; drinking too much alcohol; smoking cigarettes; air pollution; and, exposure to thousands of synthetic chemicals through the products we use, the water we drink and the food we eat.

In fact, the President's Cancer Panel report in 2009 expressed serious concern about environmental exposures explaining, "With nearly 80,000 chemicals on the market in the United States, many of which are used by millions of Americans in their daily lives and are un or understudied and largely unregulated, exposure to potential environmental carcinogens is widespread." The American Academy of Pediatrics says that babies in America are born "pre-polluted", absorbing many of these synthetic chemicals from their mothers before they are even born. Even the air we breathe is a threat with the International Agency for Research on Cancer declaring air pol-lution a "known carcinogen". In an exhaustive review of US drink-ing water, the *New York Times* concluded that many contaminants in our drinking water are not monitored by the EPA noting that, "At least 62 million Americans have been exposed since 2004 to drinking water that did not meet at least one commonly used government health guideline intended to help protect people from cancer...". According to the World Health Organization, the incidence of cancer is double in the "westernized" countries of the Americas and Europe than it is in the rest of the world and they point out that, ironically, the higher the per capita income of a country, the higher the cancer incidence. In fact, in the United States, we only have only 4.4% of the world's population but American citizens represent 7.25% of worldwide cancer deaths.

Many cancer experts believe that living in a cleaner, more natural environment is much healthier and carries less cancer risk. Yale's Yong Zhu, Ph.D., who earned his Ph.D. in molecular evolution says we should live in as natural an environment as possible adding, "I think that's the best environment for all humans...while trying to achieve balance with our modern technology that we enjoy...back to nature status, I think that's the best way to go in my personal opinion". UC San Francisco's Dr. Hiatt adds, "Basically, people have long thought that if we followed a lifestyle that was more like the way we were programed 10,000 years ago, we would probably have a lot fewer problems. I think it's a good recommendation."

Importance of Dose & Individual Variation

The dose of a carcinogen is a very important concept in cancer risk and cancer prevention. Generally, the lower the dose, the lower the risk of getting cancer and, conversely, the greater the dose the greater the risk. This applies to a range of cancer causing factors including: chemical exposures from smoking, air pollution, pesticides, drinking water that contains toxins, cosmetics, carpeting, pressed wood containing formaldehyde, insecticides, household cleaning agents, too much sun exposure, alcohol, radon in homes, radiation from medical imaging, etc. Melinda Irwin, Ph.D., Associate Professor of Chronic Disease Epidemiology and Co-Director of the Cancer Prevention and Control Program at Yale University says,

"With any kind of exposure...it's all about the dose - is it daily, weekly, monthly or yearly and how many years." Kurt Ribisl, Ph.D., Professor of Behavioral Health at the University of North Carolina, Chapel Hill says, "The amount and duration that you have smoked are very strong predictors [of health problems]...People who are fairly regular smokers and daily smokers - they are the people who experience the greatest health problems." Albert Cunningham, Ph.D., Associate Professor of Public Health at the University of Louisville and an expert in Environmental and Occupational Health adds, "There is a difference if you are exposed to a chemical for five minutes one day as opposed to eight hours a day for 20 years of your life." Tim Byers, M.D., M.P.H., Associate Dean of Cancer Prevention and Control at the University of Colorado Cancer Center points out that, "When it comes to environmental carcinogens, it's all about dose...I would just as soon not have any potentially carcinogenic chemicals in my body but I do know that at extremely low doses the body detoxifies these chemicals in a generic fashion...".

The problem when it comes to dose when you are trying to protect yourself and your family is, "How much of an exposure is safe?" That is a particularly difficult question given that there is a wide variation between individuals in terms of how well you, as an individual, can process potentially harmful environmental exposures. In fact, there is no single answer that applies to everyone since we are all so different in terms of the strength of our immune system, genetics, etc. Angeline Andrew, Ph.D., a Molecular Epidemiologist and Assistant Professor of Community and Family Medicine at the Geisel School of Medicine at Dartmouth Medical School says, "There are differences in susceptibility to different chemicals. Some people experience harmful effects at a lower dose than others so that an exposure that might not harm one person might be carcinogenic or harmful to somebody else." Dean Hosgood, Ph.D., M.P.H., at Albert Einstein College of Medicine adds:

There is a saying in toxicology that the dose makes the poison...meaning there are a tremendous amount of exposures in our life and they are not all going to be harmful and even some that are potentially harmful can be metabolized and excreted by our body...There are a tremendous amount of compensatory mechanisms in our body that can deal with harmful exposures. But who is to say at what point do the mechanisms become overburdened and what happens if you continue to have exposures...It comes down to not only the exposure and the dose of the exposure but also how your body is able to respond. How efficient are your compensatory mechanisms? Are you able to metabolize that exposure? Are you able to excrete it rapidly enough so it is not a harmful exposure to you...which varies from individual to individual.

University of Kentucky's Susan Arnold, M.D. adds, "Some people clear the DNA damage well whereas others don't...All of the risks and toxins from exposures matter but it also matters whether you can process and clear that stuff out of your body."

3

Case for Prevention

Given the life-threatening nature of many cancers, the challenges facing cancer treatment, our individual differences and the belief by cancer experts that environment and lifestyle play a major role in the development of most cancers, many cancer experts feel that, as a nation, we are not putting enough emphasis on cancer prevention and need to do much more in that regard. Elena Reyes, Ph.D., Associate Professor and Director of Behavioral Medicine at Florida State University says, "What goes to the core of this is a systemic change the entire country needs to make...lifestyle changes...". Keith Wailoo, Ph.D., Professor at the Woodrow Wilson School of Public Affairs at Princeton University states, "It is generally true that at all levels of research we have tended to focus on treatment and less and less on prevention." UC Berkeley's Luoping Zhang, Ph.D. explains, "I really think that in our fight against cancer for the last 30 or 40 years, there has been too much focus on cancer treatment and not enough on cancer prevention." East Carolina's Dr. Paul Walker adds, "If America was really committed to tobacco cessation, really committed to a lifestyle of exercise, then that would greatly reduce cancer so much better than any therapy." Robert Amato, D.O., Professor of Oncology at the University of Texas Medical School and Chief of the Division of Oncology at Memorial Hermann Cancer Center adds, "I think, absolutely, we fail as a society at putting in the resources to promote preventive care...". University of Tennessee's John Bell, M.D. says, "I do not believe we invest enough as a nation on cancer prevention." Dale Shepard, M.D., Ph.D., a medical oncologist with the Cleveland Clinic asks, "Can we prevent a lot more cancers? Absolutely." Thomas Sellers, Ph.D., M.P.H., Professor of Epidemiology at the Moffit Cancer Center explains:

> Nobody wants to pay for prevention. We have a health care system that has been historically focused on fixing people when they are broken rather than keeping people healthy. It is far cheaper to focus on prevention and maybe now with the Affordable Care Act we are seeing the tide shift to a greater emphasis on prevention and early detection and promoting health.

Oklahoma State University's Rashmi Kaul, Ph.D. adds, "If we spent more on prevention and education, we would be better off. We are only spending one dollar on education and prevention for every thousand dollars on treatment." As the President's Cancer Panel noted, "It is more effective to prevent disease than to treat it...". While cancer has some unique risk factors, some of the same risk factors that increase your chances of getting cancer apply to heart disease as well including: being overweight or obese; having a poor diet; drinking too much alcohol; and, lack of exercise. UC San Diego's John Kellogg Parsons, M.D. says, "When I talk to my patients, I tell them the things that are healthy for our hearts, in our everyday living, also tend to be things that can help us fight cancer." By exercising, eating nutritious food, not drinking alcohol at all or in moderation and exercising almost every day, people minimize their risk for the top two killers in America – cancer and heart disease. In addition, for people who accept the premise advocated by cancer experts that cancer prevention strategies have merit, then one of those strategies should be to try to reduce potentially harmful environmental exposures, such as synthetic chemicals, to themselves and their families as much as possible which will involve a real commitment on their part.

How much prevention one wishes to practice is an individual decision that will vary from person to person. People who have already been diagnosed with cancer or have a family history would probably be well advised to aggressively practice a wide range of cancer prevention measures that will be discussed in detail in later chapters. Given that the lifetime risk of cancer is one out of three for women and one out of two for men, probably everybody should practice some level of cancer prevention. Peter Lance, M.D., Chief Cancer Prevention and Control Officer at the University of Arizona says:

> Everybody is at risk for cancer and the average risk person, that is, somebody who has not been identified by some other condition that predisposes to cancer or having a family history of a particular kind of cancer, then the common sense things we already know now about a healthy lifestyle are the most important things to do. The earlier in life that one can start with these healthy lifestyles, the better.

Joshua Muscat, Ph.D., an Epidemiologist and Professor of Health Science at the Penn State Cancer Institute says if you diligently live a healthy life such as eating healthy, maintaining a healthy body weight, don't smoke, etc. and "if you can do all those things compared to people who can only do one or two of those things, your lifespan may be 10 to 15 years longer on average."

Prevention & Cancer Survivors

In fact, cancer experts say that the same healthy behaviors that can prevent cancer in the first place can also help to prevent recurrence and improve outcomes in patients who have already been diagnosed with cancer. Paul Walker, M.D., Director of Oncology at the Brady School of Medicine at East Carolina University says, "If you look at the benefit of exercise, in reducing...the recurrence of cancer...exercise even reduces development of lung cancer." Yale School of Medicine's Yawei Zhang, M.D., Ph.D. M.P.H., says that it is important for cancer patients to live as healthy a life as possible and reduce potential toxic and carcinogenic exposures adding, "Environmental risk factors that relate to the development of cancer also relate to the prognosis of the disease." Melinda Sothern, Ph.D., Professor of Behavioral and Community Health Sciences and Exercise Physiologist at Louisiana State University adds, "There are huge benefits to increasing physical activity...There are also studies that show that physical activity improves relapse, cancer remission." University of Tennessee's John Bell, M.D. says, "Control the controllable. Do the things that you can personally do by making healthy lifestyle choices that maximize your chance of both prolonging your life as well as prolonging the quality of your life...". Peter Shields, M.D., a medical oncologist and Deputy Director of the James Cancer Center at Ohio State University explains:

> The same recommendations regarding cancer prevention apply to many patients who are going to be cancer survivors...What I will say to all of them is, 'Look, I don't know that this will really impact your cancer from coming back at some time in the future but I know that you've got, in your body, cells set up to get cancer so you have proven that you are susceptible in one way or another. So now it is doubly important to follow the recommendations that we know in terms of a healthy lifestyle, exercise, all of those things. There is data that shows that people who follow those healthy lifestyles do better.'

Melissa Davis, Ph.D., Assistant Professor of Genetics at the University of Georgia says:

> For people who have already had cancer, this becomes even more important because what we have established is something in your environment has triggered your predisposition or there is something that you have been exposed to that has caused this...You definitely have to change something about your environment...The hope here is that even if you

have been exposed to something in your environment, even if it's just your lifestyle, these modifications can reverse themselves if you simply make the change - if you remove the exposure and we have data that shows this molecularly.

UC San Diego's Gordon Saxe, M.D., Ph.D. adds:

> We have pretty good evidence right now that if breast cancer patients lose weight, they are going to reduce their risk of relapse...Components of weight loss are improving diet and increasing physical activity - clearly, there is support for that...There are also numerous, numerous cases, case histories, case reports of patients who have had even advanced malignancies that have been able to stop them from growing, and sometimes reverse them, through diet and lifestyle changes...Obviously, there's no guarantee for anybody who has cancer that diet and lifestyle, they're not a cure...But I do think it's possible, if you look at a population of patients with cancer, if we can instruct them, help them to make sustained healthy, diet and lifestyle changes, that in the population as a whole, on average, we will see a slowing of the progression of the rate of cancer. Maybe for some people, the cancer will stop growing and for a smaller group, but an important group, we may actually see reversal of cancers... Cancer prevention is not just before the tumor develops, even after cancer is in place, if we prevent its progression, essentially we starve the cancer of what's needed to cause it to grow, we are doing something that's a very safe way of addressing the cancer that a person already has in their body.

Epigenetics & Trans-generational Epigenetics

The case for cancer prevention for everyone is further strengthened by the emerging field of Epigenetics, which involves gene expression that influences whether our cells grow normally or as cancer cells. Cindy Battie, Ph.D., Professor of Public Health at the University of North Florida explains:

> It is only in the last decade when we have really started to understand Epigenetics...which you can change the expression of a gene without changing the [genetic] sequence...we now know that environment affects these epigenetic markers... and it is really revolutionizing the field...I think, in many ways of how environment influences cancer.

Yale University's Yong Zhu, Ph.D. adds, "Epigenetic factors might play a more important role than genetic factors... ". University of Georgia's Melissa Davis, Ph.D. notes, "Epigenetics is the hopeful part of the story...If you just remove the chemical, the exposure, your cells will eventually find their way back to a normal state so you can prevent tumors from happening if you change now...epigenetic changes are completely reversible." Yawei Zhang, M.D., Ph.D. M.P.H., Associate Professor of Cancer Epidemiology at the Yale School of Medicine adds, "You can't change your genetics but you can definitely change your epigenetics." Michael Skinner, Ph.D., Professor of Biochemistry at Washington State University says, "Epigenetics... probably has an equally important role as genetics and the thing about these epigenetic processes is they can be dramatically influenced by environmental exposures...". Thomas Jefferson University's Dr. McMahon adds:

> Epigenetics is linked to genetics because it affects how our DNA is expressed...It's a new field in terms of our molecular understanding of it. So much more has to be discovered before we really understand the epigenetic patterns...As we learn more about it, it will certainly contribute to cancer prevention and we will be able to predict what environmental carcinogens work via the epigenetic mechanisms to cause changes in genes that could cause cancer.

Increasingly, cancer experts are also exploring the new field of trans-generational epigenetics which is not as well established as epigenetics but is beginning to gain ground. It suggests that it might be helpful for young people to keep in mind that how they live now can affect not only their children in the future but their grandchildren. It also holds that parents hand down both genetic and epigenetic characteristics to their children. William Hendry, Ph.D., Professor and Chair of the Department of Biological Sciences at Wichita State University explains:

> Regarding epigenetics, a classic story is that during World War II there was a phenomenon called the Dutch famine. A large part of the population there was in starvation… Researchers went back and studied not only the children but the second and third generations of the progeny of that group and they have obesity problems, they have diabetes, etc. It seems that their epigenetics were reprogramed…and that was passed on to their progeny. Subpopulations being exposed to their environment has affected not only the individuals exposed but sometimes the following generations.

Washington State University's Michael Skinner, Ph.D. says:

> The thing about these epigenetic processes is they can be dramatically influenced by environmental exposures… whereas the sequence of the DNA cannot be changed by environmental exposures…What I would do is, in terms of counseling an individual… what they need to do affects their offspring and grandchildren as well…is called epigenetic trans generational inheritance. That is a form of non-genetic inheritance…Essentially, when you reproduce, you are going to pass it onto the next generation…It turns out, if you look at the sperm, it is actually carrying the altered epigenome, there's these chemical modifications in those sperm that are passed from generation to generation.

Carlos Sonnenschein, M.D., Professor of Integrative Physiology and Pathobiology at Tufts University School of Medicine adds, "Trans-generational epigenetics is real which you may be prone to have but you can have a positive impact on your epigenetic imprinting by reducing exposures [to carcinogens]." UC San Diego's Dr. Saxe concludes, "Cancer prevention has a far greater potential than most of us realize for addressing the problem of cancer."

% of Cancers that are Preventable

Indeed, many experts believe that a significant percentage of cancers are preventable. Dean Hosgood, Ph.D., M.P.H., at Albert Einstein College of Medicine says:

> The World Health Organization came out with a very detailed review that was done by about 500 of the world's leading experts and they concluded...that a large number of cancers are from preventable sources...I would agree that there are many things that individuals can do to minimize the risk of cancer...

The estimates of preventable cancers vary a bit as one might expect since some people have more opportunities to implement cancer prevention strategies than others. For example, it is well known among cancer experts that wealthier, better educated people have more knowledge and resources to follow cancer prevention recommendations than poor people with lower education. The following represent a range of estimates of the percentages of cancers that are preventable. The World Health Organization says at least one-third of cancers are preventable. Linda Birnbaum, Ph.D., Director of the National Institute of Environmental Health Science, a division of the National Institutes of Health, says, "While you can't change your genes, you can change your environment...cancers related to environmental exposures range from about one third to about two thirds of all cancers and I am defining environmental very broadly there to include nutrition, smoking, alcohol and anything that is not specifically a genetic cause." Laura Vanderberg, Ph.D., Professor of Environmental Health at University of Massachusetts School of Public Health Sciences adds, "I would think that somewhere in the range of 50 to 60% is justifiable." Graham Coditz, M.D., Dr. P.H., Associate Director of Prevention and Control at the Siteman Cancer Center at Barnes-Jewish Hospital points out that, "For about 20 years, we have been saying that the percentage of preventable cancers is in the 50 to 60% range and the evidence for that keeps getting stronger and stronger." Clemson University's Charlie Wei, Ph.D. says, "I believe that 70% of cancers or more are preventable." Pebbles Fagan, Ph.D., M.P.H., Associate Professor of Prevention and Control at the University of Hawaii Cancer Center says, "75% of cancers can be prevented." Carlos Sonnenschein, M.D. adds, "Most of the cancers that we get both as adults and children are preventable... In my view, 80% of the cancers are preventable." Anthony Alberg, Ph.D., M.P.H., Professor of Public Health at the Medical University of South Carolina breaks it down saying:

> Cigarette smoking is a cause of at least 30% of all cancer deaths. Infections are thought to cause 18% of all cancers... Alcohol is thought to account for 3% of all cancers...Air pollution and other environmental factors about 2%...Sunshine about 3% of cancers...Occupational exposures account for about another 4%...That takes us up to about 60% of cancers being preventable...Preventable cancers may be higher than that because of factors associated with obesity and lack of physical activity...Up to 90 to 95% of cancers could be attributable to what we would broadly refer to as environmental causes...There are some factors that appear to be controllable at the individual level and some of the societal level where progressive public policy to come into play...air pollution is an example.

Two Good Examples of Effective Cancer Prevention – Smoking Cessation & Vaccines

Two examples of cancer prevention efforts in the United States illustrate the potential effectiveness of cancer prevention strategies. The first has been the development of two vaccines that can now prevent certain cancers caused by the Human Papilloma Virus and Hepatitis B. Thomas Kensler, Ph.D., Professor of Cancer Pharmacology and Cancer Prevention at the University of Pittsburgh explains, "Cervical cancers and liver cancers are eminently preventable ones with the universal vaccination programs." The second good example of cancer prevention is the dramatic reduction of smoking rates in recent decades in the US that was followed by a reduction in lung cancer cases. Susan Mayne, Ph.D., Professor of Epidemiology and Associate Director of the Yale Cancer Center says, "Smoking rates used to be well over 50% in the United States - we have made tremendous gains in tobacco control...8 million Americans avoided premature deaths as a result of tobacco control efforts following the Surgeon General's report in 1964."

Section II

Modifiable Risk Factors for Cancer

4

Tobacco Use

Risk Stratification

As you begin to plan your own personalized cancer prevention program, consider everything you have learned about cancer prevention and the opinions of experts. Certainly consider that some risks are so well established and do so much harm to public health that they should be at the top of your list. University of Pittsburgh's Thomas Kensler, Ph.D., notes, "Well over half of human cancers should be preventable - we know the causes, we know what to do… There is a cascade of risks, big risks and smaller risks." For example, smoking is the number one cause of preventable death in the US and throughout the world. If you do not smoke, don't start but if you do, try to quit. Susan Mayne, Ph.D., Professor of Epidemiology and Associate Director of the Yale Cancer Center says in terms of cancer prevention, "I would emphasize the big two factors that we know are really strongly related to human cancer and accounts for a large proportion of human cancer and those are tobacco smoking and being overweight or obese which is reflecting diet as well as physical activity…". Smoking, overweight or obesity and lack of exercise are all especially important because they are risk factors for cancer and heart disease. Proper nutrition has protective features against cancer and must also be very high on the list as do vaccines against HPV and Hepatitis B which prevent cervical and liver cancers respectively.

Acknowledging that smoking, overweight/obesity and regular exercise are very important for good health is not to suggest that you should in any way ignore the other cancer risks. The President's Cancer Panel, American Academy of Pediatrics, and many cancer experts have been warning of the dangers of the largely untested 80,000 chemicals in our environment. The International Agency on Caner Research has declared air pollution to be a "known carcinogen" as noted earlier. An effective cancer prevention program should include a plan to eliminate as many potentially harmful environmental exposures as possible. While public health experts think in terms of public policy that addresses the most people, you as an individual have to protect yourself and your family from as many risks as possible. Radon, sunburn, excessive alcohol, synthetic chemicals in water, air and food cause cancer and collectively take the lives of hundreds of thousands of Americans each year and millions worldwide. Just because they do not kill as many people as smoking does not mean they will not impact you or someone in your family. The primary reason to even mention stratifying risks is for people who want to practice minimal cancer prevention efforts perhaps because they have no known family history of cancer and are willing to accept the risks to their health and that of their families, if any, that go with such a decision. Those people should focus on the top few items in the previous paragraph. For all others who wish to take a more aggressive approach to protect themselves and their families against the substantial lifetime risk of cancer in the US noted earlier - take appropriate action to address all of the known and reasonable likely risk factors.

Don't Smoke

Dangers of Smoking

Smoking increases the risk of getting cancer by 20 to 30 times that of a non-smoker. While smoking has declined in the US, almost one out five Americans still smokes which is much too high and contributes to hundreds of thousands of American deaths each year and millions worldwide. John Neuberger, Dr. P.H., an Epidemiologist and Professor of Preventative Medicine and Public Health at the University of Kansas Medical Center, says that in the US, "The hardcore smokers are not quitting yet...Cigars and pipes also pose a substantial [cancer] risk." Penn State's Joshua Muscat, Ph.D. says, "Smokers are actively breathing in a complex mixture of well over 100 toxins, several carcinogens and breathing this stuff deeply, it's like the worst possible poison you can think of...". University of North Carolina, Chapel Hill's Kurt Ribisl, Ph.D. notes that smoking is the number one cause of premature death adding that, "In the US, tobacco use causes 440,000 deaths per year from lung cancer and heart disease...". Dean Hosgood, Ph.D., M.P.H., at Albert Einstein College of Medicine says, "Of all the tobacco studies, there have not been studies that have shown any safe levels from what I understand." UC San Diego's John Kellogg Parsons, M.D. points out that, "Smoking not only causes cancer but emphysema, a very debilitating lung disease, as well as cardiovascular disease." Smoking not only increases the risk of lung cancer which is usually fatal, but other types of cancers as well. Carlos Crespo, Ph.D., Professor of Community Health at Portland State University says, "Smoking increases your risk for the four leading causes of death: cancer, heart disease, stroke and diseases of the lung. Smoking is related to all four of them." Anthony Shield, M.D., Associate Director of the Barbara Ann Karmanos Cancer Institute at Wayne State University adds, "There are numerous other cancers that people don't necessarily think about that are associated with smoking such as head and neck, tongue, lip, esophagus, stomach, pancreas, bladder, cervix and occasionally leukemia...and despite that, way too many Americans continue to smoke."

Addictive nature of nicotine

Tobacco use is not the free choice made by adults that the tobacco companies would like people to believe. Bob Mc Caffry,

M.D., Director of Oklahoma Tobacco Research Center says, "We know that 75% of smokers want to quit...". In addition, the vast majority of smokers begin as children or adolescents. Tobacco companies market to and addict children to nicotine, one of the most addictive substances known to man, which is totally contrary to free choice as most people understand it. Bill Fields, Ph.D., M.S., Professor of Epidemiology at the University of Iowa explains, "When you are younger, all those factors that may come in, this is in the future and I'll quit someday...that addiction may overwhelm any free choice they may have." Dartmouth Medical School's Angeline Andrew, Ph.D., a Molecular Epidemiologist and Assistant Professor of Community and Family Medicine at the Geisel School of Medicine at Dartmouth Medical School adds, "Approximately 20% of high school students have smoked recently despite the fact that we know that it's a huge risk factor [for cancer]." University of Arizona's Peter Lance, M.D. says, "It is critically important to recognize that tobacco is an incredibly addictive substance...".

Roy Baumeister, Ph.D., Professor of Psychology at Florida State University and Author of the New York Times Best Seller, "Willpower: Rediscovering the Greatest Human Strength" explains:

> For people who have other psychological problems, then smoking becomes a way for them to cope...Even though smoking cigarettes is a stimulant, a lot of people report that it relaxes them...One argument is that once you get addicted and you haven't had a cigarette, you start to go into a small withdrawal state and having a cigarette feels like it's relaxing because it gets rid of the withdrawal state.

University of Massachusetts' Laura Vanderberg, Ph.D. adds that, "Smoking is easy to control until you start doing it and then you're addicted to it." Lorraine Reitzel, Ph.D., Professor of Psychology at the University of Iowa says:

Once kids get into smoking, they get addicted to it and some of the choice about smoking is taken out of the picture...There are actually physiological changes in the brain such that your body requires a certain amount of nicotine in order for a person to feel like they're functioning at the right level. So, if a regular smoker has not had a dose in a little while of nicotine via a cigarette, you are going to start to feel a little anxious, some physiological symptoms that tells you 'I need another cigarette'...

If You Don't Smoke, Do Not Start – That Goes for E-Cigarettes as Well

Given the highly addictive nature of nicotine, the best strategy for any individual is to never start smoking. This message needs to be reinforced by all adults with all young people including from parents, teachers, clergy, community and national leaders. It should be an integral part of every health curriculum in every school in the US and throughout the world. E-cigarettes are relatively new on the US market and are highly controversial. They are essentially flavored, nicotine delivery devices that use water vapor combined with attractive flavors instead of smoke from tobacco. Even though they do not have the carcinogens from burning tobacco, they do deliver highly addictive nicotine to their users and the danger is that if these become widespread, children who observe adolescents or adults using them may emulate that behavior and start using regular cigarettes to obtain their "fix" of nicotine. On the other hand, if e-cigarettes are carefully controlled such as by prescription for people who are trying to quit smoking, then a limited use of them in the United States may be worthy of consideration. George Yu, Ph.D., Associate Professor of Molecular and Cellular Biology at Clemson University relates his own personal experience with e-cigarettes saying:

I used to smoke and then the hospital placed a ban on tobacco use on the whole medical campus which prompted me to quit with the help of e-cigarettes...There are various types of filters that can adjust the amount of nicotine you take in so I just gradually reduced the amount of nicotine while I was trying to quit and then the last couple of weeks while I was using e-cigarettes there was no nicotine being delivered but it was the psychological effect [that helped]...

The use of e-cigarettes might be a worthy option to help people to quit smoking but only if used in the privacy or their own homes and never in front of children. America must be very diligent not to let companies selling e-cigarettes set back American public health interests after all of the hard fought gains against tobacco use.

If You Smoke, Try to Quit

If you smoke and are able to quit, you will reduce your risk of lung cancer, heart disease and be healthier in many ways. The Siteman Cancer Center's Graham Coditz, M.D. says, "If you smoke cigarettes, cut down and stop since that's the fastest way to get carcinogens into your body." Unfortunately, however, the truth is, that because of the addictive nature of nicotine, quitting will not be easy and smokers will likely make a number of attempts before they are successful. University of Colorado's Tim Byers, M.D., M.P.H. reminds people that, "If you failed [to quit smoking] a few times - congratulations. That means you're on the right path. People who succeed have always failed a few times before they succeed." If you cannot quit on your own, seek outside help through a formal program, group support or individual counseling.

For example, Bob Mc Caffry, M.D., Director of Oklahoma Tobacco Research Center suggests using the 'Quit Line' offered by many states saying, "Only about 2% to 5% of smokers who try to quit without outside help are successful...We actually have had a fair percentage of smokers in Oklahoma who have utilized the Quit

Line [with a much better quit rate]". Kurt Ribisl, Ph.D. adds, "Seek help. Every state has a 'quit line'...and those help people quit - people can walk through the different steps and help them find a quit date, help them deal with the triggers...". Dean Hosgood, Ph.D., M.P.H., at Albert Einstein College of Medicine says of those trying to quit, "Support groups and healthy workplace initiatives can help people to stick with it." Kim Pulvers, Ph.D., Professor of Psychology at California State University, San Marcos says individual counseling combined with nicotine replacement can be an effective strategy noting, "There is a biological and psychological reason that people keep smoking...Nicotine replacement...may help with the biological piece...One-on-one therapy can help the individual...Some of the best programs include a counseling component...". Dr. Ribisl points out that people with mental health problems especially need counseling to help them quit smoking saying:

> Among people who have some type of mental health problem, we've done a bad job - their quit rates have not dropped nearly as well...40% of all cigarettes are consumed by people who have some type of mental health problem... schizophrenics have an 80% smoking rate as opposed to 18% for the general adult population.

Also, do not allow yourself to be exposed to second hand smoking by others which is a known cancer risk. Louisiana State University's Edward Trapido, Ph.D. asks, "Do you live with smokers? Do you spend time around smokers? The most important thing that somebody can do is avoid exposure to tobacco smoke one way or another." Virginia Commonwealth University's David Wheeler, Ph.D. adds, "Avoid exposure to secondhand smoke including public places where people are smoking if you are not a smoker." The Siteman Cancer Center's Graham Coditz, M.D. says, "If you live with someone who smokes, get them to smoke outdoors and stop as fast as they can. Avoid second-hand smoke."

The "Partnership" between US Tobacco Companies that Market to Children & US Government Policies that Contribute to Childhood Smoking in Developing Nations

In spite of declines in smoking in the United States, the *Journal of the American Medical Association* points out that for the first time in human history, we are approaching one billion smokers on the planet. The World Health Organization and others say that smoking will contribute significantly to the projected increase in worldwide cancer incidence. The vast majority of smokers start before they are even adults and the tobacco industry has a long history of marketing their products to children – a tactic that they widely used in the US prior to losing lawsuits to states' attorney generals. Wallace Akerley, M.D., a medical oncologist and Director of Thoracic Oncology at the Huntsman Cancer Institute at the University of Utah explains:

> For a tobacco company, if you are going to expose someone or create an addict [to nicotine in cigarettes], it would be much greater to create an addict who is five years old who can smoke for 70 years versus creating an addict who is 70 years old already who doesn't have much time left...There is no question in my mind they have been advertising to young individuals forever.

University of Arizona's Peter Lance, M.D. says, "Nicotine is one of the most addictive substances there is and kicking the habit once people have started is a major problem and it's not something that developing countries are equipped to do."

Yet, tobacco companies have now exported their marketing tactics to children in developing nations preying on many of the world's most vulnerable where there is little or no protection forthcoming from their governments. Dr. Peter Lance says, "There is a huge problem in the developing world with tobacco which is a very cheap product so tobacco companies are undoubtedly exploiting that." Dr. Tim Byers adds, "It's just shameful what's going on in developing countries...The tobacco companies, not just the American companies, are using really shameless approaches for marketing tobacco." Marc Schenker, M.D., M.P.H., Professor and Chair, Department of Public Health Science and Medicine at the University of California, Davis says of the marketing of tobacco products to children in developing countries, "It's all true. It's despicable what tobacco companies do."

The tobacco companies have an important "partner" in the form of the United States government because of its failure to join all of its allies around the world to ratify an important treaty aimed to reduce tobacco use. University of Hawaii's Pebbles Fagan, Ph.D., M.P.H. explains, "There is a treaty called the Framework Convention on Tobacco Control. It was the first health treaty that was ever developed at a global level...to reduce tobacco use at a global level." More than just the US allies, over 175 countries have signed onto the treaty. Among the relative few that are not supporting this most important worldwide public health initiative in addition to the United States are Cuba, Haiti, Somalia, El Salvador and South Sudan – not exactly stellar company for the leader of the free world. In fact, the US government opposed key provisions that would protect children in developing countries such as bans on the distribution of free tobacco samples, limitations concerning tobacco advertising and requirements for warning labels to be written in the language where the tobacco products are being sold. In addition, the US government promotes smoking in developing nations through its trade policies. Graham Coditz, M.D., Dr. P.H., Associate Director of Prevention and Control at the Siteman Cancer Center at Barnes-Jewish Hospital explains:

> Some of our trade agreements facilitate the trade of tobacco to countries that may not have had very high smoking rates in the past...We have done an amazingly good job of exporting

smoking to parts of the world that were not smoking and they are now replicating the epidemic of lung cancer...

Comparable to the US government's disregard for the health of children in developing countries as demonstrated through its public policy positions is China which owns the tobacco companies there, generates tax revenues but is facing a major epidemic of male smokers on its hands. Dr. Peter Lance, M.D. says, "China has a monumental tobacco problem that is just waiting, it is a tsunami that's going to come...there is going to be a huge epidemic of tobacco-related disease in China that is coming down the pike in the next coming decades." At least in China, their ownership of tobacco companies is out in the open whereas in the US, the tobacco industry's "ownership" of many American politicians in Congress is much more covert. Tufts University School of Medicine's Carlos Sonnenschein, M.D. suggests that, "People should press their representatives in Congress to do the right things...The issue is that these representatives are in the pockets of the big industries." Karl Kelsey, M.D., M.P.H., Professor of Community Health and Director of the Center for Environmental Health at Brown University says, "One of the big roles of the government is to protect people from products that are dangerous or hazardous...". Unfortunately, the US, Chinese and other governments that have not taken steps to prevent children from starting to smoke have failed in meeting this most basic responsibility.

Public Policy Approaches to Smoking

First, the United States government needs to promptly stop its policies that contribute to the massive export of tobacco that is combined with marketing to children in developing nations and its "partnership" with tobacco companies that will doom many millions of children to poor health and premature death. It is imperative that the US ratify the Framework Convention on Tobacco Control and become a global leader in this most important initiative to protect children's health around the world. It should also change its trade policies and use its influence to protect children in developing nations from the predatory American tobacco company practices that prey on them. Laura Anderko, Ph.D., R.N., Cancer Epidemiologist and Fellow at the Center for Social Justice at Georgetown University adds, "I would encourage people to be informed consumers but also to push hard legislatively whether it's a call or shooting at 30 second email to say we need stronger policies."

Here at home, although we have made progress with smoking in the US, almost one in five still smoke and we need some renewed initiatives to get those rates down as near to zero as possible. University of North Carolina, Chapel Hill's Kurt Ribisl, Ph.D. outlines the approaches:

> Believe it or not, tobacco use is not that hard to change. We can cut it in half in the US easily simply by putting into place what we know works. We have a lot of evidence from places like California, New York, Florida and other states that have implemented tobacco control programs that have had dramatic reductions in smoking rates...It's pretty easy to get people to quit smoking or not to start - what's hard is to get politicians to agree to put in place effective policies that do that. The number one thing we can do is increase the price of tobacco products which is typically done through taxation...It causes kids not to start, it causes current users to smoke less or quit. In countries where tobacco use is high, cigarettes are ridiculously cheap. The second thing is strong tobacco free air laws – ban smoking in workplaces, bars, restaurants and so forth...The third one is banning or restricting tobacco advertising and marketing. Fourth is promoting [smoking] cessation - giving people quit lines, access to medications that help people quit.

University of Hawaii's Pebbles Fagan, Ph.D., M.P.H. echoes the importance of smoking bans in public places noting:

Adopting smoke-free environments is important. In Hawaii we have, right here in the Honolulu area, smoke-free beaches, for example, to reduce people's exposure to that environmental pollutant because we know there are...chemicals in cigarettes with many carcinogens and people, including small babies, can be harmed by someone else's smoking behavior.

Advertising of tobacco products continues to be a problem that prompts people to smoke. Lorraine Reitzel, Ph.D., Professor of Psychology at the University of Iowa points out that:

These tobacco retail outlets that increases the urge to smoke and that can make people who are trying to quit smoking more vulnerable when they go in there to buy gas or something because they see advertisements for tobacco and that might engender an urge to smoke and make them purchase it...and now there's advertising on television for e-cigarettes which is alarming to me.

5

Overweight, Obesity and Nutrition

The Problem

Obesity is a major contributor to cancer and other diseases in the developed and developing world. Overweight and obesity are major contributors to many major chronic illnesses including three major ones in the US – cancer, heart disease and diabetes – and contributes to premature death. Susan Mayne, Ph.D., Professor of Epidemiology and Associate Director of the Yale Cancer Center says, "The data are unbelievably strong linking overweight and obesity with increased incidence of many, many cancers including the most common cancers...The excess risk for obesity approaches a doubling of cancer risk if you look at all cancers combined....". Stanford University's Alice Whittemore, Ph.D. says, "Keep your body weight under control because being overweight is a risk factor for certain cancers...". Joseph Ahlander, Ph.D., Assistant Professor of Biology at Northeastern State University adds, "If we are talking about obesity as a major cause of preventable disease, it is number two right behind smoking." Paul Dale, M.D., Chief of Surgical Oncology at the Ellis Fischel Cancer Center and Professor of Medical Research at the University of Missouri School of Medicine adds, "A lot of cancer risk seems to be related to our diet and what we eat here in the Western world compared to other parts of the world where there are certain types of cancers that are less prevalent...". Oklahoma State University's Rashmi Kaul, Ph.D. points out that, "Fat tissues produce excess amounts of estrogen and these high levels of estrogen are the risk factor for breast cancer, endometrial cancer, liver cancer, colon cancer and thyroid cancer...".

Overweight and obesity is not just a problem in the US, but has become a major problem of global proportions. Where underweight was once one of the biggest health problems in developing countries, it is now obesity. University of Colorado's Tim Byers, M.D., M.P.H. notes, "Obesity and overweight is not just a problem in the developed world like the US but is a pandemic...its everywhere." University of Arizona's Peter Lance, M.D. says, "The Western lifestyle is introduced and in a relatively short period of time you see these cancer risks increasing." This does not bode well for ourselves, our children or our grandchildren. University of Kentucky College of Medicine's Nancy Schoenberg, Ph.D. explains that for the first time in many years in America, "...life expectancy is declining, my children's generation is expected to have less years of life than my generation and that's a real concern...speculation is around overweight, obesity and lack of physical activity." The problem is so bad in the US that today, two-thirds of Americans are either overweight or obese. In addition to all the physical health problems, obesity is also closely tied to depression. Dr. Schoenberg notes, "There is a very compelling evidence of the association between obesity, overweight and depression...". It also contributes to poor productivity and time away from work. In other words, overweight and obesity are major problems on multiple fronts.

Causes of Obesity

Genetics and Environment

If we are to have any chance of turning around the obesity epidemic in America and thereby making more progress against common chronic diseases including cancer, heart disease and diabetes, we need to understand the causes. It is important to note that overweight and obesity are a relatively new problem in the US and throughout the world caused by multiple factors including an abundance of affordable, caloric dense, unhealthy food that is marketed by food companies combined with a sedentary lifestyle. As noted earlier in the discussion about human evolution, throughout most of human history, people were physically active hunter gatherers and then for most of the last 10,000 years were physically active farmers or other physically active occupations. In addition, food was scarce and our bodies evolved with a fat storage mechanism which was a protective factor for times of severe food shortage to protect against starvation. That trait often does not serve us well in developed countries where food is usually plentiful. Walter Willet, M.D., Dr. P.H., Professor of Epidemiology and Nutrition and Chair of the Department of Nutrition at the Harvard School of Public Health explains:

> The reasons that it is so hard for us to lose weight are complex and there is no single reason. Clearly, there are strong biological mechanisms that tend to encourage us to eat and those have been built in by evolutionary forces because for most of our existence...we have been threatened by starvation and inadequate calories rather than too many calories. So, we have mechanisms that tend to promote eating and storage of fat. That doesn't mean that it is inevitable that we become obese. Second, we have created an environment that is very conducive to overeating.

Furthermore, for the vast majority of human history we did not have all of the office jobs and televisions to sit in front of for hours on end every day. In the past, people worked longer hours than today with less leisure time and discretionary income to purchase and consume all of the excess, unhealthy food and soft drinks we consume today. The problem has gotten much worse in recent decades with the heavy marketing of unhealthy foods to children, of which one in six in America is now obese. Dr. Willet adds, "...if we just go back to 1960, overweight and obesity was far less of a problem than they are now - the obesity rates in adults were only about one third of what we have now."

In addition to a biological role from evolution, genetics also plays a role in obesity. Clemson's George Yu, Ph.D. says, "Genetics does play some role in obesity and some people just more easily get overweight and once you become overweight, it is harder to lose." Paul Walker, M.D., Director of Oncology at the Brady School of Medicine at East Carolina University adds:

> For those of us who tend to have non-obese genes, I think it's very easy to think, 'Oh it's only a matter of willpower' but I think it's clear that it is not...Why can some people eat all they want with no problems, and others, you feel like, 'Golly, at Christmas time how did I gain these 3 pounds?'

Washington State University's Michael Skinner, Ph.D. adds:

> In the 1950s, the obesity rate was 3%. Today, it is over 35%. What we are doing is inducing a susceptibility to develop obesity. So if there's two individuals, one is susceptible and one that is not, given exactly the same diet, exactly the same exercise, exactly the same nutrition, basically, the one that is susceptible will develop obesity. Clearly, lifestyle will contribute to the onset of obesity but the susceptibilities that develop appear to be induced by genetic and epigenetic hereditary factors.

Tracey Ledoux, Ph.D., Assistant Professor of Nutrition at the University of Houston who specializes in the treatment of obesity adds, "Hereditary factors for children increase if one or both parents are overweight or obese...". Indeed, if one parent is obese, their offspring has a 25% risk of being genetically predisposed to obesity and if both parents are obese, the risk increases to 80%. However, in addition to genetics, environment contributes to that phenomenon in those households. Louisiana State University's Edward Trapido, Ph.D. says, "People who have grown up, for example, in a family where both parents are obese, are going to be used to an eating pattern that is considered excessive." Furthermore, the problem becomes self-perpetuating due to obese people marrying each other. Harvard University's Walter Willet, M.D., Dr. P.H. explains, "There will be something that we call sort of the 'mating factor' as thin people tend to marry other thin people and fat people tend to marry fat people so that will concentrate fat disposing genes somewhat…".

Experts agree that genetics and environment both play a role in obesity. Cindy Battie, Ph.D., Professor of Public Health at the University of North Florida says, "It's very hard to lose weight. It's genetics, its environment…it's socioeconomic status…it's a combination….and food is a pleasure, it's family, it's cultural." However, not all experts agree as to what percentage of overweight and obesity can be attributed to environment vs. genetics. Dr. Ledoux says, "…[it is estimated] that 70% of that tendency to be overweight or obese comes from genetic factors…". Bruce Ames, Ph.D., Professor Emeritus of Nutrition and Metabolism at the University of California, Berkeley counters, "There is a genetic obesity too but that is relatively small percentage of obese people…If it was a result of genetics, we would have had it forever but it just shot up in recent years." Northeastern State University's Joseph Ahlander, Ph.D. adds, "If you look at obesity over just the last several decades, the genetics of the population hasn't really changed yet obesity has increased two to threefold in the United States which is clearly the result of environment and lifestyle factors…". Dr. Willet points out that:

> Genetics do play some role in people who will become obese but usually we find an interaction between genetics and the environment. In Japan, Sweden and France, it's not that they are genetically different than we are because people from those places come to the United States and they get fat

like other people here do. Also, genetics cannot explain the increase in obesity that we have had here in the US in the last 40 years. If we really had the optimal environment, we probably would only be at only 2% or 3% of people who would be obese.

Jamie Ard, M.D., Co-director of the Weight Management Center at Wake Forest Baptist Medical Center adds:

The majority of what we see in terms of obesity in this day and age is primarily dictated by excess calorie intake and not enough physical activity...There are some people who have a genetic propensity for gaining weight...The genetic contribution to obesity is probably somewhere around 5% or 6%...Only about 6% of the weight that an adult achieves is attributed to genetics and the other 94% or 95% of that is accounted for by lifestyle and behavioral issues. Some people just have to work a little bit harder, make a few more sacrifices...Practically speaking, for most people, their destiny is in their own hands.

According to the American Journal of Clinical Nutrition, "The mechanisms contributing to obesity are complex and involve the interplay of behavioral components with hormonal, genetic and metabolic processes, obesity is largely viewed as a lifestyle dependent condition." Erin Eaton, Ph.D., Associate Professor of Biology at Francis Marion University comments on the biology of it explaining:

Some people have a higher or lower metabolism...and the more active you are, the higher the metabolism is and the more you burn off the 'fuel'...It's not necessarily the number of fat cells but rather the amount of triglycerides and the size of the fat cells...When you lose fat you are burning the triglycerides and the fat cells get smaller but as you're storing them it's literally the fat globules that cause the cells to get bigger.

Emotional & Psychological Factors Related to Overeating and Obesity

There are also significant emotional and psychological aspects related to obesity. Jean Kristeller, Ph.D., Professor Emeritus of Psychology at Indiana State University explains:

> I rarely ever see anybody who does not have emotional and psychological associations with their eating. You do, I do, everybody does. Because food has meaning. 'Why did you want chocolate cake? Well, because, let me think, why did I want it? Oh yeah, that was my grandmother's best cake. I just love that kind of cake'. That is a psychological attachment that is stronger than, 'I just like chocolate'...One of the early studies that I actually did was around simply asking people about how they related to food, what were their eating patterns, what did they see as some of the issues that they had. 80% of the people said they ate for emotional reasons...You have had a bad day, you want 'comfort food'... Normal people eat food for all kinds of emotional reasons... but there is a continuum and some people binge eat...about 20% to 30% of obese individuals have binge eating disorder.

Binge eating is defined as eating large amounts of food continuously for up to 2 two hours at least once per week and feeling out of control and regretful that it happens.

Florida State University's Elena Reyes, Ph.D. adds, "Most patients who are treated, both adults and children, for obesity also have a comorbid mental disorder." Overeating to the point of obesity does not seem rational but people often do irrational things. Steven Barger, Ph.D., Professor of Psychology at Northern Arizona University says, "The way we think about it as thoughtful psychologists is that we think people are rational, thoughtful, reflective in terms of these decisions and I think the data suggests that we are none of those things in that context." Dieticians who work with obese patients often have to confront emotional and psychological issues with their patients and will frequently make referrals to counselors. Yale Cancer Center's Maura Harrigan, M.S., R.D. explains:

> Someone who has had a lifetime struggle with their weight, that means that something they have been dealing with through their adult life often has origins in childhood and childhood eating patterns. So emotionally, what you're dealing with is someone who has struggled with this for a long time and, from a dietitian's viewpoint, to have what I call a 'dieters mentality', a black and white, good and bad view of food. Their relationship with food becomes, I hate to use the word 'distorted', but there is a real disconnect between actual hunger and feeling full and the actual amount of food that they eat. They have kind of lost that connection of eating to appetite, responding to hunger cues and stopping eating when they are full. So the counseling component when dealing with people who have had a lifelong struggle with their weight is really going at those eating behaviors...You cannot ignore depression...I have made many a referral to, when I seen their depression is in the way, to counseling or a psychiatrist...the majority of patients require counseling.

The emotional roller coaster that some people ride can contribute to weight regain after successfully losing some weight. John Pierce, Ph.D., Professor of Family and Preventative Medicine and Co-Leader of the Cancer Prevention Program at the Moores Cancer Center at the University of California, San Diego says of obese people who lose weight:

> The majority put it back on. It's like smoking. It's habitual... It's very hard to change these lifetime habits that you have developed, particularly in the adolescent years...so you have stress and you go to the fridge. People who are obese have

had a lifetime of taking in more calories than they need and that's how they handle their lives. They have 'mood foods'. If they're in a bad mood, they eat...People behave themselves for a long time and then all of a sudden 'pig out' and the 'pigging out' can undo three weeks of good work in a single session. The problem is they went so well for so long and then something happens and they get into a mood and they eat so many calories it's not funny. That's not genetics – that's a behavioral eating problem...

Poor Nutrition in America and its Links to Obesity & Cancer

For anyone who wants to lose weight, it is much more important to consider that all experts agree that there is a genetic and environmental component rather than getting hung up on which of those two factors plays a larger role. You cannot control the genes you inherited, but you can definitely do something about your environment and lifestyle. A good starting point is to consider that most Americans have poor diets which contributes to overweight, obesity and cancer. Certain foods are believed to have protective qualities against cancer such as cruciferous vegetables including broccoli, cauliflower, cabbage, cress, bok choy, kale, brussel spouts, turnip roots and mustard seeds. Robert Hiatt, M.D., Ph.D., Chair, Department of Epidemiology at the University of California, San Francisco says, "Diets containing fruits and vegetables can protect against cancer." Jeff Bland, Ph.D., former Professor of Nutritional Biochemistry at the University of Puget Sound and President of the Personalized Lifestyle Medicine Institute explains:

> There are certain dietary principles that augment the body's detoxification processes such as cruciferous vegetables like broccoli, cauliflower, brussel sprouts, and cabbage that have these phytochemicals in them that are known to help the body's detoxification processes with carcinogenic chemicals. One should consider things that relate to foods that

have adequate levels of fiber that promotes proper gastro-intestinal function that are known to be anti-carcinogenic.

Robert Turesky, Ph.D., Professor of Medicinal Chemistry and expert in food and nutrition at the University of Minnesota echoes those sentiments saying, "You should have a varied diet with plenty of antioxidants, cruciferous vegetables." Mark Doescher, M.D., Professor of Family Medicine and Program Leader in Cancer Health Disparities at the University of Oklahoma Health Sciences Center says, "I try to get people to eat a nutrient rich diet including lots of fruits and vegetables and cut back on the high salt, sugar, carbohydrates...".

Studies show that the majority of Americans do not get the 30 essential nutrients recommended by dietary experts and the federal government. UC Berkeley's Bruce Ames, Ph.D. explains:

> The American diet is a disaster. We are starving for vitamins and minerals and eating too much refined food that's full of calories but it sort of empty calories...In the US population, the following percentage of people are below the Estimated Average Requirements for various nutrients – the official measure of nutrient adequacy in the US – even with supplements it's a disaster: vitamin D - 70%; vitamin E- 60%; magnesium - 45%; calcium - 38%; vitamin K - 35%; vitamin A - 34%; vitamin C - 25%; zinc - 8%; vitamin B6 - 8%; folic acid - 8%. When you look at those numbers you realize practically everybody is deficient in one thing or another...

A poor diet not only denies people the protective qualities from healthy foods like cruciferous vegetables, but it also contributes to overweight and obesity. There is a theory that when people are missing essential nutrients in their diets, they tend to eat more because, even though they are eating a lot of high caloric, unhealthy food, their bodies are starving for the essential nutrients it needs thus overriding the body's mechanism that tells it that it is satiated or full. As a result, they still feel hungry and continue to overeat. Harvard University's Walter Willet, M.D., Dr. P.H. acknowledges this theory but says more research is needed, "There is a hypotheses that has not been clearly confirmed. First of all, it is very true that Americans are, on average, way far away from optimal diets. In the total population only about 5% meet the current dietary guidelines...". In addition, some foods make you feel fuller than others which helps to cut down on overeating. The *European Journal of Clinical Nutrition* noted that, for example, if you eat 300 calories of doughnuts, you would be more likely to still feel hungry than if you ate 300 calories of oatmeal cereal. UC Berkeley's Bruce Ames, Ph.D. says, "We have done 17 clinical trials or so in people and given them lots of minerals and vitamins and fiber and it makes people less hungry."

Health experts say the American diet is too high in fats, red meats, refined sugars, salt and calories which contribute to our high cancer rates. John Erdman, Ph.D., Professor of Food Science and Human Nutrition at the University of Illinois says, "Eating foods that we all know are healthy and avoiding those that are unhealthy reduces the risk of cancer." UC San Francisco's Dr. Hiatt says, "There is good evidence that the consumption of red meat is associated with colorectal cancer and eating less red meat is a good idea." Joshua Muscat, Ph.D., an Epidemiologist and Professor of Health Science at the Penn State Cancer Institute explains:

Cancer rates in China and Japan in the early 20th century were 20% that of the United States. Why is that? It's probably because the diets in those Asian countries were dramatically different from Western diets. A diet in Japan which is primarily plant-based, fish based, that's probably the major reason why...The reason we know it's nutrition because people have migrated from Japan and other Asian countries to the United States and then their cancer rates go up dramatically...They started consuming westernized high caloric diets. Now that they have been here for 30 or 40 years, the migrants have the same rates of cancer as other European or American citizens.

The Role of Marketing by Food Companies, Culture, Affordability & Poverty

Why do Americans and increasingly other developed and developing countries around the world have such poor diets? There are several primary reasons. One of those is cultural with certain traditions around food that varies between countries. Yale School of Medicine's Yawei Zhang, M.D., Ph.D., M.P.H. explains that:

> In a Chinese diet, we hardly ever eat desserts but here desserts are a major thing after a meal. During the meal, you should have already gotten the nutrients that you need while the desserts are just carbohydrates and when they get into the body if you don't need that energy, it immediately gets converted to fat...

Harvard University's Dr. Willet adds:

> In Japan and Sweden, the prevalence of obesity among women is only about 5% or 6% whereas here it is around 35 to 40% and those are not poor countries. People can afford to buy all the food they want. They don't get fat like we do. The environment there is very different. Culturally, there is much more emphasis on quality rather than quantity of food and they are not supposed to eat until their full but are supposed to eat until almost full...

In addition to cultural influences, we are surrounded by delicious, affordable and fattening food. Brian Wansink, Ph.D., Director of the Cornell Food and Brand Lab and Professor of Consumer Behavior at Cornell University says, "If you compare us now in 2014 to 1960, food is much more accessible, attractive and affordable. In 1960 the family spent about 26% of its income on food, now we spent about 6% on food...It's also more attractive - more flavors, more packaging ...". Indeed, food companies have mastered the art of marketing unhealthy products to us while making them appear to be very appealing. UC San Diego's John Pierce, Ph.D. says, "I think the problem is marketing. We market the hell out of things and package them in ways with enormous amounts of calories." Dr. Willet elaborates:

> There is a food environment in the US basically related to the fact that every food company, every food retailer is out there to get us to eat more of their product and they are competing with each other to get us to eat more of their products. They do lots of research and have invested billions of dollars to maximize the seductiveness of the products in terms of flavor, texture, color and then spend a huge amount on marketing and packaging it in an attractive, seductive way too and place it everywhere so there's food in front of us almost all the time. Then there's the advertisements themselves through every media you can name and even more seductive media, interactive, Internet, programs that get us into brand loyalty and this marketing has gotten more powerful year-by-year because of the research so that the imbalance between our native defenses to help us control our eating and the power of marketing and food promotion gets more unequal and especially problematic for kids who have less awareness, less consciousness and are more susceptible...

Some psychologists study the impact of food marketing on consumer behavior. Steven Barger, Ph.D., Professor of Psychology at Northern Arizona University says:

> ...if you think about people in the United States, we are all exposed to almost trillions of dollars of food advertising,

marketing, etc...The food marketers and the people in the grocery stores, they have armadas of evidence and they are constantly testing approaches to get people to buy stuff and we do...If you think about the amount in the advertising budget...you think you are in charge of your universe and you make choices that are your choices but in fact you are incorrect. The choices you make are driven by those kinds of marketing activities. They wouldn't do them if they didn't work.

Indeed, food companies that market unhealthy food to children are contributing to an obesity epidemic among children. Given that one of six American children are now obese, University of Arizona's Peter Lance, M.D. expresses his concern saying, "We really need to grapple with the problem that we have in our developed society with more and more children becoming obese." Lynn Panton, Ph.D., Associate Professor at Florida State University explains, "We have to start young because it's very difficult once you are older, and you have these bad habits...We have to educate our children...about the proper food choices. It is very difficult once you're older to change those behaviors." As a result, many of these children will be facing a variety of health problems in the future including cancers, heart disease and diabetes.

Some American food and beverage companies have taken a page out of the tobacco companies' playbook and are now exporting their unhealthy products and all the marketing that goes along with them to children in developing countries. Yale's Yawei Zhang, M.D., Ph.D., M.P.H. explains, "In the past, you never heard about obesity issues in China. But now...the worst childhood obesity is not in the United States, it's in China. Obesity and diabetes in China is increasing rapidly...The most profitable junk food restaurants are in China. McDonald's and fried chicken, they're everywhere...". Harvard University's Walter Willet, M.D., Dr. P.H. says, "In Japan, there is some of the Western promotion with McDonald's and other places and it's starting to show up in some of the kids with some increase in obesity…". In an investigative report aired on PBS, children in poor countries were shown to be marketing targets with a goal of getting them to drink large bottles of Coca Cola and Pepsi Cola along with a wide range of other unhealthy snacks contributing to an obesity epidemic in those countries. The caffeine in those and other soft drinks have mildly addictive properties which help get children hooked on them. UC San Diego's John Pierce, Ph.D. says, "We have converted people from drinking water to drinking sodas." Dr. Peter Lance adds:

> As we look around the world, we see within a generation, a short period of time, from my father to me or whatever, in one generation cancer risk has changed. For instance, colorectal cancer used to be a much less common problem in Japan, but then with the McDonald's golden arches, within one generation or two generations, suddenly colorectal cancer rates increased to what we find in Western countries.

In spite of heavy criticism of food companies that are marketing unhealthy foods to children, most have not shown much of an interest in changing. Why? The sad truth is that the wealthy shareholders and executives of these companies, like the tobacco companies, are becoming even wealthier by peddling the seeds of poor health to children worldwide. University of California San Diego's Gordon Saxe, M.D., Ph.D. says, "…whether it's resistance from the food industry that is sluggish in providing the healthy alternatives…from what I've seen, there is a huge amount of resistance which does not make me very optimistic…". Virginia Commonwealth University's David Wheeler, Ph.D. says, "There are powerful forces out there that don't want you to change." Cornell University's Brian Wansink, Ph.D. adds, "Hoping that the food industrial complex is going to change, it's going to be a long wait."

Poverty and low education also contributes to a poor diet which contributes to overweight and obesity with a commensurate cancer risk. In some poor communities, it is difficult to find a grocery store with really healthy alternatives. University of Kentucky College of Medicine's Nancy Schoenberg, Ph.D. says that, "A good portion of our nation lives in food deserts - both urban and rural - if you've got an environment that really doesn't have a great offering of fresh fruits and vegetables, or affordable high quality foods then it becomes a real challenge to have a good eating pattern."

Fast food companies have capitalized on this fact by placing and marketing their unhealthy products in poor communities contributing to the obesity problems among the poor. Lorraine Reitzel, Ph.D., Professor of Psychology at the University of Iowa says studies show, "That there are a lot of fast food restaurants in areas that have lower socioeconomic status…and the more fast food you eat, the higher your body mass index…and if you don't have a lot of money and you know that fast food is cheap then it becomes a particularly attractive option for you." Yale Cancer Center's Maura Harrigan, M.S., R.D. says, "A person can easily consume their total daily calories, 2000 to 2200 calories, in one meal at a fast food place." Cindy Battie, Ph.D., Professor of Public Health at the University of North Florida points out, "When you go to McDonald's, what do you see? Calories. If you are an uneducated person, how do you know how many calories you should be taking in…if you live in certain areas, and you don't have a car, you can't get good food."

Our Busy American Lifestyle, Overweight & Obesity

Many Americans are often on the run with things like jobs and their children and they often do not take the time to cook nutritious meals for the family. Penn State's Joshua Muscat, Ph.D. explains:

> The problem is that maintaining proper body weight is difficult to do with the Western lifestyle. This has been known for a long time. People are working and it's hard to cook and

prepare fresh foods, it's very easy to go out and buy high caloric foods and this creates a problem. It's kind of built-in, to a certain degree, with our lifestyles.

University of Iowa's Dr. Reitzel adds:

A lot of the mechanisms that underlie behaviors like eating foods that aren't so good for us are things like stress, being under a time crunch, being under a lot of pressure. We have to jam so much into a single day that making the food choices like eating fast food as opposed to going to the grocery store and buying fresh vegetables and then going home and cooking them and then feeding your family - sometimes is not really an option because people are working more than 40 hours a week. By the time they get in their car, pick up the baby, get home and have a bunch of things to do, they don't really have the time even it is the way they want to eat.

Potential Solutions to Poor Nutrition, Overweight & Obesity

Losing Weight – Be Realistic About the Challenges Ahead

We have a major problem pertaining to the ability of overweight and obese people to lose weight and keep it off. Experts agree that the data is absolutely and indisputably compelling that the vast majority of them who try to lose weight do not succeed in the long term. Many can lose weight in the short term, such as six months or up to a year, but then gain it back – sometimes weighing more than when they started the diet. Worse yet, many try over and over again with no success. University of Houston's Tracey Ledoux, Ph.D. says, "People would lose weight and then regain it...70 to 90% of people who lose weight regain it within five years, most within the first year...". Thomas Sellers, Ph.D., M.P.H., Professor of Epidemiology at the Moffit Cancer Center says, "One of the problems with diets, rather than change in lifestyle, is that people only lose weight for a short duration and then people go back to their usual diet which caused them to gain the excess weight in the first place...". Florida State University's Roy Baumeister, Ph.D. says, "What one usually hears is that is that about 90 to 95% of people who diet gain back all the weight within a couple years and often they gain back even more than they lost." David Just, Ph.D., Director of the Cornell Center for Behavioral Economics for Child Nutrition Programs adds, "People who keep weight off for like five years is well below 10% and probably even lower than 5%...it's really tough...". Barbara McCahan, Ph.D., Professor of Health and Physical Education at Plymouth State University Center for Active Living says, "Because the statistics have been so grim in terms of people trying to lose weight, I personally have turned my efforts and energy into better understanding why and applying good health and exercise psychology...". Portland State University's Carlos Crespo, Ph.D. points out that, "It's hard to gain weight for 10 or 20 years and then pretend that in one month you are going to lose it all and keep it off...".

For morbidly obese people, it is even worse. They have little chance of losing most weight much less keeping it off. Joseph Aloi, M.D., Director of the Sterlitz Diabetes Center at the Eastern Virginia Medical School in Norfolk says, "I can think of 10 people in my 20 year career who lost 100 pounds or more and kept it off in the long term without surgery."

Why is it so difficult to lose weight and keep it off? University of Houston's Tracey Ledoux, Ph.D., Assistant Professor of Nutrition at the University of Houston who specializes in the treatment of obesity explains:

> Research and clinical experience over and over and over and over again shows that simply getting on a diet, starting to follow a meal plan is not going to be a sustainable weight loss program...You will probably lose some weight on the

front end but it will not be something that they will be able to maintain for the long haul. There are small segments of the population that can maintain weight loss but in my experience people do not want to hear that, people want an easy fix and they have doubt when you start getting too negative about it...I like to talk to people about how all-encompassing this is. It's not just about eating behaviors and exercise, it's also about their behavior outside of that - their grocery shopping behaviors, their restaurant behaviors and emotional management, their stress management, their sleep habits, caffeine consumption - it's really a holistic kind of an approach that they really need to alter - sort of an overhaul of their entire lifestyle. I don't think people really get how all-encompassing it is to make these changes in a sustainable way...People want to lose it and they think they will be the exception...and this time will be different...'I was wrong about trying it [the last diet that failed] that way'...Many of the people that I see are repeaters...and this one time will be different than every other time that they have tried to lose weight in the past. There is this motivation, hope and euphoria as they jump into this new plan of how things are going to be but then slowly, slowly, slowly begin to settle back down to where they started from and the weight starts to come back on.

Jean Kristeller, Ph.D., Professor Emeritus of Psychology at Indiana State University adds:

Most of the diet approaches, with some exceptions, try to simplify people's eating patterns to a degree that is quite unrealistic. In other words, they are very structured diets that say, 'Eat this, don't eat that' and the issue is that people end up learning that pattern - the 1,200 calorie diet, for example, but don't learn how to maneuver through all of the challenges of eating... They are going to go back to the eating patterns that they had before. When I have asked, 'What happened? How did you start gaining that weight back?' 'Well, I went to a birthday party and I had a piece of cake...'. They are seeing that as a failure rather than, 'I can have a piece of cake, I just can't have half a cake' and they interpret that as a breakdown in their resolve, they throw up their hands and say 'I just can't do this. Why should I try'...Very slowly what happens is that older patterns that are over-determined by their family, by their environment, by all of those food choices they face every day, just show up again...

Harvard University's Walter Willet, M.D., Dr. P.H. says physical health problems can contribute to the problem of weight loss as well explaining:

It's hard to be physically active if you are obese as there is more to carry around and often times people have already started to develop complications that make it harder to be active such as arthritis, diabetes, cardiovascular disease so there are higher barriers than there were prior to the development of the obesity.

What makes it especially difficult for people to lose weight is the constant temptations of when others are eating fattening food around them including their own families or when food is ever-present at social events. Lorraine Reitzel, Ph.D. says, "Often, risk behaviors occur within families. As a family, we cook together, we eat the same foods, we do the same things, we are physically active or we are not physically active, so it is often helpful if we can get... support from a husband or wife...". Just as emotional and psychological issues can contribute to gaining weight in the first place, so it can contribute too to regaining it. Joel Hughes, Ph.D., Professor of Psychology at Kent State University says:

Weight is incredibly hard to control and part of that is a psychological explanation. For example, it's hard to control your environment, you can control yourself to a certain degree, but you can't dictate what kind of environment you are going to be in so sometimes our efforts at behavior change is swimming upstream against the environment that you are in. For example, we have a lot of easy access to high calorie food in America and as other countries have improved distribution of food, they start to have obesity problems too... It is absolutely true that some people have psychological problems like depression, let's say, that makes it hard to obey the things that they are supposed to do. Loneliness is another factor - there is some research that shows that being socially isolated makes the cookie taste better. Social rejection seems to increase the value of nonsocial rewards... However, most people don't have psychological problems and yet most people are overweight.

Potential Solutions – What to Do to Improve Your Nutrition and Lose Weight if Needed

When searching for solutions to the overweight and obesity problem, experts say that we should stop thinking about short term diets and start thinking about permanent and sustainable lifestyle changes that are characterized by really healthy eating and exercise that is almost daily. It will be challenging. Mark Dignan, Ph.D., Director of the Prevention Research Center at the University of Kentucky College of Medicine says:

> I think the path between having information and knowledge and changing your behavior and maintaining it is a long, twisting, tortuous path...It's hard for somebody to decide to try to lose weight, make a lifestyle change and then to maintain that over a long period of time. It is very difficult

to do unless you make a completely fundamental change in your life in the way you do things.

Gary Meadows, Ph.D., Professor of Pharmaceutical Science at Washington State University adds:

> First of all, we ought to get rid of the word 'dieting' because in order to maintain a weight loss you have to have a lifestyle change. That means watching the calories, writing down what you eat, exercising, it needs to be a lifestyle change, not something you do in the short term. It's what you do in the long term and that's not easy. Also, dieting usually involves depriving yourself of certain types of foods and I don't think that's healthy because then when you're deprived and you all of a sudden go off diet, you want a treat. I think you need to do it in steps. It's a long-term, rest of your life lifestyle change. In my opinion, that's the only way you can maintain the weight loss.

In addition, experts say avoid fad diets. Penn State's Joshua Muscat, Ph.D. explains:

> Obesity is an important risk factor for breast cancer and colorectal cancer...It has been known for a long time that dieting does not work...There have been many popular diets that have been recommended over the last 20 to 30 years... and by and large these diets tend not to work...The weight loss industry has a long history and track record of this, it has not been successful...

It does not help people to look at pictures of models and hope that is what they will look like after they lose weight. That is not what most of us look like or should even strive toward. Plymouth State University's Barbara McCahan, Ph.D. explains:

If you look on the cover of any woman's health magazine, you will see a skinny long-haired woman scantily clad and that's the way we are all supposed to be. That's the message. We are inundated with messages that you must diet, you must diet, you must be thin...We need to resist those messages and be joyful about who we are, what we are regardless of our size... The more we can love ourselves and move into the kinds of behavior that care for our body well - I think that makes us healthier regardless of our size...

Pay close attention to what you eat and what's in it. University of Hawaii's Pebbles Fagan, Ph.D., M.P.H. says:

Read food labels, know what you are consuming and how many calories are in the food that you are purchasing...You have to start by doing an assessment of your behavior. What are you consuming? Are you drinking a lot of sweet, sugary beverages? Are you consuming lots of carbohydrates like breads? Then begin your behavior change. Setting goals is really important...Over this particular time period, this is what I want to accomplish.

John Spangler, M.D., M.S., a Family Medicine physician at Wake Forest Baptist Medical Center, recommends:

...small changes, cut out the soda for example, no in between meal snacks, cut down on portion sizes...cut back 500 calories per day...pushing yourself away at the table at the end of the meal...drinking water between each bite... Having social support is absolutely crucial...The key is to find someone who is going to cheer you on...someone who is not going to shame you when you slip up but will encourage you...

If you do need to snack, experts recommend healthy snacks like fruit.

While setting weight loss goals is important, the goal must also be realistic. According to a study published by the *Journal of Clinical Diabetes*, most people who join weight loss programs often want to set their goals at 20 – 30% loss of their body weight. Based on research, this has not been realistic for most people so set your weight loss goal realistically – when you hit it, you can get more aggressive. Northern Arizona University's Steven Barger, Ph.D. says, "Humans have what we call unrealistically optimistic beliefs about a lot of things." David LaPorte, Ph.D., Professor of Psychology at Indiana University of Pennsylvania adds:

> It's hard to lose weight…If I am overweight and I set my goal to be normal weight, to look like people on TV ads, newsprint or anywhere else, I am not going to make it probably because that is an unrealistic goal for most people who are obese. But from a health standpoint, losing some weight… they will be a whole lot healthier.

Joel Hughes, Ph.D., Professor of Psychology at Kent State University says, "As difficult as smoking is to change, obesity is even worse - it's the Holy Grail…One of the things that we fight psychologically is that people's expectations for how much weight they are going to lose is almost always more that is realistic." Yale Cancer Center's Maura Harrigan, M.S., R.D. adds:

> …the goal does not have to be getting to normal BMI…that's not how dieticians work – the goal is to get a 5% reduction from the weight you are starting with…What a lot of people don't realize is that a 5% weight loss is considered clinically significant - you will reap the medical benefits in terms of a healthier blood pressure, managing your blood glucose levels, your heart will benefit, your kidneys will benefit and

when people hear that they will often say, 'That's it? I can do that'.

UC San Diego's John Pierce, Ph.D. asks of people who set unrealistic weight loss goals:

> When were you last at that weight? It's probably when they were teenagers. How many times have you gone on diets to try to do this? Is it really an achievable goal? If you haven't lost five or 10 pounds [and kept it off], how are you going to lose 100 pounds? How is that going to happen? An achievable goal is based on what you have done before and can you do a little better. If you shoot for the moon, all you do is destroy yourself efficacy. You should not be setting a goal that there is no possibility you can do...If an obese person has a BMI of 35, the best we will be able to do is get them down to 33 in the long run.

Harvard University's Walter Willet, M.D., Dr. P.H. says:

> A lot of times people have unrealistic expectations, particularly for someone who has had excess weight for quite a while...It's difficult to lose 20%, 30% or 40% of weight... Some people are successful so I would not say it's impossible...but you should feel very good about yourself if you could even lose 5% and keep it off...It's almost impossible to get back to where you were at the beginning and in part even the bones will have gotten bigger because they respond to a larger weight to carry around and that's not something easily reversed but from a health standpoint there are major benefits to a 5% or 10% weight loss.

When trying to lose weight and maintain the weight loss, eat healthy which, as Cornell's David Just, Ph.D. says, means always "keep your head in the game". That means learning what a healthy diet looks like and then adapting it as a lifetime change. Jean Kristeller, Ph.D., Professor Emeritus of Psychology at Indiana State University explains:

> I would sort of raise a challenge regarding what I call 'mindless eating' - sitting down and eating snacks in front of the television...People have the ability to change habits and change patterns over a period of time. It can happen but it is a slow process and you need to have an attitude about doing it – it is by no means short term and takes into account, 'I am going to have challenges. I'm going to have some ups and downs...I am going to have a new relationship to my eating that is permanent not just for the time being, for the moment or just for the next six months while I lose this weight'.

It is important to understand that a healthy diet can help you to feel satiated or full. If you do not feel hungry all the time, you will eat less. Many nutrition experts believe that a largely plant-based diet similar to the Mediterranean Diet meets the test of a really healthy, nutritious diet. Harvard University's Dr. Willet explains:

> One of the most successful randomized trials was a diet conducted in Israel...it compared a Mediterranean diet with another diet low in fat and at the end of two years...the low-fat diet participants regained much of their weight while the Mediterranean diet participants kept most of their weight off even after four years when they went back and checked with the participants. What they found was a way of eating that was satisfying with a good variety that they could incorporate into their usual way of living and that's really the most important ingredient. Extreme diets are not sustainable over the long run...Mediterranean diet includes whole grains, fruits and vegetables and there are many, many ways to put that together.

In addition to helping you lose weight and keeping it off, a healthy diet helps with disease prevention. Ann Schwartz, Ph.D., Deputy Center Director at the Barbara Ann Karmanos Cancer Institute at Wayne State University adds, "Having a Mediterranean type diet with lots of fruits and vegetables is something that could help prevent cancer...". Moffit Cancer Center's Thomas Sellers, Ph.D., M.P.H. says, "Diet is obviously important. The Mediterranean Diet seems to be most healthy in terms of not only cancer [prevention] but other disease risks."

In addition to lots of fruits and vegetables, a Mediterranean diet can include small amounts of lean meat and/or fish. US News and World Reports now ranks different popular diets just as it has ranked colleges, universities and hospitals for years. The Mediterranean Diet ranks high as do some other similar diets. Jay Thomas Sutliffe, Ph.D., Associate Professor of Public Health at Northern Arizona University says that globally, "...there are seven pockets of people who live to be 100 years old with vitality with regularity and one of the across-the-board life practices is that they have primarily a plant-based diet with small amounts of animal food that we are talking about." UC San Diego's Gordon Saxe, M.D., Ph.D. asks, "Do you have to be vegan to be healthy? No, we really can't distinguish between the level of a diet that, let's say, 95% plant-based and 5%, a small bit of food, condiment level use of healthy meat like grass-fed or wild fish, from a purely vegan diet."

In addition to a healthy diet and given the fact that most Americans are missing so many nutrients form their diets, consideration should be given to taking a vitamin and mineral supplement but experts advise against loading up on any one vitamin which can actually be harmful. John Kellogg Parsons, M.D., Associate Professor at the University of California, San Diego Moores Comprehensive Cancer Center explains:

There is a low end of the spectrum when you don't get enough vitamins and that's bad for you. The middle, healthy, range is where you get just the right amount of vitamins and it is fine to take supplements to keep you in the 'just right' range but there used to be a belief that more is better with respect to vitamins and that there were certain vitamins that you could take a lot of such as vitamin C to try to prevent colds and flu's but the more definitive research has shown that it is not the case and that too much of anything is not necessarily a good thing...There is some research now that even suggests that if you take too many of these supplements it can cause problems and actually increase the potential for you to get a particular kind of cancer.

Rubina Haque, Ph.D., R.D., Associate Professor of Nutrition and Dietetics at Eastern Michigan University adds, "If you take all the right foods consistently, you would not need a vitamin supplement but because most of us don't eat the fruits and vegetables every day and do not get the right amount of dietary fiber...a simple vitamin supplement is all one needs...".

Getting sufficient vitamins and minerals is critically important to our health. UC Berkeley's Bruce Ames, Ph.D. says:

We find that when your body is low on vitamins and minerals, it accelerates diseases of aging so I think this will be the big opportunity in cancer prevention...Every big disease has links to obesity - brain dysfunction, you name it and it increases with obesity...Vitamins are dirt cheap, we could solve this problem...I would advise everybody to take a multi-vitamin/ mineral pill and be sure it has vitamin D because you need 20 minutes or so of sunshine to make your vitamin D.

Harvard University's Walter Willet, M.D., Dr. P.H. concurs adding, "I think it's reasonable for most people to take a multi-vitamin, multi-mineral that has a little bit of extra vitamin D." John Erdman, Ph.D., Professor of Food Science and Human Nutrition at the University of Illinois explains:

> There are some chronically low level of nutrients in our diet such as vitamin A, zinc, iron, copper, a number of things that are chronically low in our diet and we don't seem to be doing better. Why? Because we're not eating a variety of foods including high amounts of fruits and vegetables. We are also not getting enough fiber because we are not eating enough whole grains. We just don't choose the right kinds of foods. Colorectal cancer is very high because we are not getting enough fiber like the kind that comes in whole grain cereals...There is certainly nothing wrong with a one a day supplement as long as people do not use it as a crutch, for example, 'I do not have a good diet so I'm going to take a vitamin supplement now and I will be okay'. That is a very invalid thinking and strategy because they are not getting all the good bioactive nutrients in food - it does not replace a good diet. The chemical in a vitamin pill is either as good or better. Centrum, as an example, that is a company that has put millions and millions of dollars into research to assure that they have bioavailable components in their vitamin pills...Some of the fly-by-night vitamin companies who sell their vitamins for pennies, you can't be sure that the vitamins are bioavailable [percent of a nutrient compound that can be readily absorbed by your body].

Dragos Albinescu, Ph.D., Associate Professor of Chemistry at Northeastern State University adds:

> Vitamins are chemicals. Any chemical at some point has toxicity including water. If you drink too much water, you can die because it disorganizes your electrolyte balance and your body stops functioning. It's the same with any

chemical. If you take too much vitamin D or A or C, you may reach the toxicity level...Vitamin supplements are good if they are taken in moderation to compensate for insufficient dietary intake of vitamins...very few people do have a balanced diet...Eating a nutritious diet is best. For example, even though the vitamin C in a vitamin supplement is the same chemically as it is in an orange, the vitamin C that you get from the orange has better bioavailability which means the same vitamin C that is taken from a natural source is better absorbed in your system then it is from the synthetic version...The synthetic vitamin C is absorbed to some extent but you need to take more of it to reach the same level of bio availability than you would from getting it from a natural source like an orange.

Being alert to eating consistently healthy or "keeping your head in the game" also means that, given our environment with all of its temptations, you always need to be on guard working to avoid those temptations and remove them in your own home. David Just, Ph.D., Director of the Cornell Center for Behavioral Economics for Child Nutrition Programs says:

Changing your diet requires you to put your head in the game always. It's this high cognitive cost that you're facing all the time and really what behavioral economics does is it teaches us that a lot of the decisions that we make about what we are going to eat are really because of what's around us...What that means is I can restructure things that don't require that level of effort so that when we are in the moment and I don't have my head in the game, that I can actually do something a little healthier. If I have my cereal sitting out on the counter, is that where it is easier for me to keep it and every time I walk through that kitchen...maybe I'm hungry and maybe I'll grab a handful of cereal...Find a place to put that cereal like in a cupboard is not something that requires me to think all day, it's not like a diet, it's a very simple act...Now every time I walk into the kitchen, I don't have that thought...If I replaced that cereal with a basket of fruit and go to the store to be sure I have fresh fruit available, now I have something triggering me that says maybe I should have some fruit. Those types of behaviors can be very sustainable and can last...

Walter Willet, M.D., Dr. P.H., Professor of Epidemiology and Nutrition and Chair of the Department of Nutrition at the Harvard School of Public Health concurs adding, "Almost everybody in America will gain weight unless they take conscious steps not to do so...".

Eat a diet rich in diversity. Henry Thompson, Ph.D., Professor of Agriculture at Colorado State University explains:

>...eat whole food products - get away from the processing, try to get away from ingredient-based food...Your mom probably told you to have a lot of variety in your diet...I don't think there's a very good understanding of how to have a botanically diverse diet so the goal is to give people the tools so that they can increase the botanical diversity of the diets that eat...By having a strategy of eating from a diverse food supply, we minimize the exposure to deleterious, harmful factors and increase the likelihood that we will get exposure to things that are good for us even if they are present in small amounts.

Mark Brick, Ph.D., Professor of Agriculture at Colorado State University adds:

>Our food choices are pretty awful with the amount of deep-fried food that we eat and the lack of diversity in food. We often limit our intake by very narrow choice of processed

foods that contain a lot of starch and sugar. If we wanted to change our diet, diversity would be the best way to do it… and less processed foods.

UC Berkeley's Bruce Ames, Ph.D. adds:

A vegetarian diet is mostly pretty good…but you do get a few vitamins from meat such as vitamin B-12 and some other things and fish turns out to be very important because you get your omega-3 fatty acids from fish…I eat fish a couple times a week…The whole trick about diet is to eat lots of different things…Fruit is very healthy – an apple a day does partially keep the doctor away - eating more fruit and nuts is very healthy and so are berries.

In addition, cut back or eliminate the sweets and excessive carbohydrates including ice cream, cakes, cookies and candy. University of Hawaii's Pebbles Fagan, Ph.D., M.P.H. says, "Replace things like chips, cookies and cakes with healthy alternatives like vegetables and fruits which becomes your new lifestyle." If you can handle eating very small amounts to satisfy your craving without eating too much and ruining your diet, that should be fine but be realistic. Some people cannot handle small amounts and it is like an addiction. Lorraine Reitzel, Ph.D., Professor of Psychology at the University of Iowa says, "There actually are a number of academics who argue that you can actually have an addiction to certain types of food - a real addiction to fat, greasy, sugar-based food." If this applies to you, with chocolate for example, eliminate it from your diet totally.

The National Institutes of Health recommends the following:

- Avoid foods that are high in fat and sugar
- Reduce how much alcohol you drink
- Avoid stress, frustration and boredom

- If you are depressed, seek treatment by a mental health professional
- Perform aerobic exercise for at least 30 minutes a day, three times a week
- Increase physical activity by walking rather than driving
- Climb stairs rather than using an elevator or escalator
- A slow weight loss of 1 or 2 pounds per week is best
- Eat 500 calories of food less every day to lose 1 pound per week
- Talk your primary care physician about weight loss and your diet

Especially for obese people, but this could apply to anyone, seek counseling help if emotional or psychological issues are standing in your way of being successful with these lifestyle changes and consider joining a high quality program that meets your budget. Jamie Ard, M.D., Co-director of the Weight Management Center at Wake Forest Baptist Medical Center explains:

> Psychological and emotional factors are really significant in overweight and obesity from the development standpoint as well as the treatment and management standpoint...A lot of people dealing with overweight and obesity are often using food as a way to manage their emotions, comfort themselves, deal with stress, so we see a lot of emotional eating, a lot of stress eating, with increased risk of depression and some other mental health challenges in individuals who are obese...If we have someone who is not managing stress well, depressed, who is using food to medicate then it is going to be a difficult challenge no matter what type of dietary approach I prescribe and what type of exercise I prescribe. Their ability to adhere to such a program will be affected by their mental health...I think that a significant majority of obese people who want to lose weight are dealing with some type of behavioral challenge and would

benefit from a series of interventions that would help them to build some necessary skills so they can apply that in the way they think about their lifestyle...For individuals who struggle with their weight over a long period of time, there are usually multiple issues that are often compounded by a complex medical history such as diabetes, sleep apnea, arthritis and other things that also make living a healthy lifestyle even harder...If a person stays engaged in the program over a long period of time, they have a better chance of long-term success...More than just a few months but really, truly for the rest of that person's life. This is really a new era that I think we are moving into where we are starting to 'get it'...

Eastern Michigan's Rubina Haque, Ph.D., R.D. adds, "Unless you make a lifetime change and learn how to eat well, the changes won't be sustainable...It takes months and years for people to really learn how to change their eating habits...".

People who try to lose weight exhibit many different characteristics, habits, behaviors and personality traits that lead to different dieting approaches and different results. Roy Baumeister, Ph.D., Professor of Psychology at Florida State University says:

Some factors that contribute to weight involve genetic predispositions and things that are beyond an individual's control...Some people are overweight because they don't eat sensibly or are just undisciplined but others are overweight because they cannot help it and no matter how much they restrict their eating, they are not able to lose weight.

For anyone trying to lose weight, it might be helpful to study the characteristics of people who have lost weight and successfully keep it off as well as the characteristics of those who were not successful. Then, perform an honest self-assessment to determine which of the two groups you most likely match up with based on your personal characteristics. In an article that was published in the *Journal of Clinical Diabetes*, the characteristics of people who did and did not successfully maintain weight loss were revealed as follows:

Characteristics of People who Experienced Early Weight Regain

Pre-treatment: older age; Mexican-American; high number of previous diets; high maximum baseline weight; frequent binge eating; all or nothing thinking; dietary disinhibition; low exercise and diet self-efficacy; low motivation; unrealistic weight loss goals; and, negative body image.

Post-treatment: early weight regain; not responding to the early weight regain; continuing of weight loss efforts; high levels of perceived hunger; dissatisfaction with level of weight loss; dietary disinhibition; frequent emotional eating; frequent binge eating; diet high in calories, fat and sugars; decreased frequency of exercise; and, TV viewing of greater than 2 to 4 hours per day.

Characteristics of People who Successfully Kept Weight Off

Post-treatment: high levels of physical activity; diets low in fats, calories and sugars; frequent self-monitoring; consistent eating habits throughout the week and year; regular consumption of breakfast; catching small slips before they turn into large weight gains; limited TV viewing; regulated emotional eating; help-seeking behavior; and, direct coping with stress and behavioral lapses.

Before starting your lifestyle changes, conduct your honest self-assessment and if you have one or more of the characteristics of the pre-treatment people group who gained weight back early, then you should consider getting professional help from a counselor who has experience working with people who are trying to lose weight or a professional program like one associated with a major medical center near you. Wake Forest's Jamie Ard, M.D. says, "We use a comprehensive team of individuals from dietitians, exercise trainers, psychologists, health behaviorists, physicians and nurses to put together a comprehensive plan." While everyone would likely benefit from using a high quality weight loss program with professional counselors and registered dieticians, for people who exhibit the characteristics of early weight regain group described above in the study published in the *Journal of Clinical Diabetes* – it's probably a must in order to be successful at long term weight loss.

There are many organizations and individuals studying potential solutions to the obesity epidemic with some promising findings. James Gurney, Ph.D., Professor of Epidemiology at the University of Memphis School of Public Health explains:

> The Robert Wood Johnson Foundation is an example of a terrific organization that is putting a lot of money into trying to educate and change factors related to obesity using a multidimensional approach...They are looking at school initiatives, they are looking at studies related to personal success, etc...There are some indications that it is letting up so hopefully we will see a receding of the rates of obesity - we have already seen a plateau. Now the question is, can we start to reduce it within coming birth cohorts and I think there are a lot of efforts to do that and I think there will continue to be.

Public Policy Role in Weight Loss and Healthy Eating

Government, communities and school systems also play an important role in improving healthy eating and reducing obesity in America. Many children do not get the kinds of food that they need at home for a variety of reasons. Often, the parents themselves do not eat right which is easy to believe given that more than half of Americans do not get the 30 essential nutrients needed as mentioned earlier. Sometimes, the children are from low socioeconomic households and the lack of money and education contributes to poor nutrition for the children. Schools can help fill the void. Cornell University's David Just, Ph.D., says we need to develop effective strategies to help children to learn to eat healthy explaining:

> At Cornell [our program for schools for children] uses the environment of the school lunch to encourage kids to choose healthier foods on their own. If we can get the kids to eat healthier, it actually lasts for a long time…I think there are some places [schools] where they do a very good job and there are certainly places I can find where they either do a poor job or they don't do any job…We've got to start marketing healthy foods and healthy lifestyles the same way high sugar cereals are marketed to kids…We have to make it socially acceptable for kids to eat healthy…Put a sticker of Elmo on apples and you get 70% of kids to choose apples. Back in the 1930s there was a survey of kids favorite food and number one was ice cream and number two was spinach because of [the famous cartoon character] Popeye [who became strong when he ate his spinach]…There's nothing inherently appealing about smoking or drinking coffee but these become popular with kids because of the way they are marketed.

The United States and other countries need to follow the lead of our neighbors to the south, Mexico, on a courageous initiative they have begun in an attempt to turn around their nation's obesity problem, which is even worse than the one in the US. They are imposing sales tax on high calorie, fattening snacks such as soft drinks and potato chips. Nancy Schoenberg, Ph.D., a medical anthropologist with the University of Kentucky College of Medicine explains:

...to change, to really have fundamental change in our society with obesity patterns requires a commitment on a lot of different levels well beyond the individual to achieve the outcome required. It requires some reining in of the food industry, some policy level changes. In other countries, for example, Mexico has a tax on sugar sweetened beverages and that tax is fairly sizable...The Mexican government decided that its citizens, which are the most obese of any nation in the world, they have to provide some guidance and some limitations on purchasing because they are at tremendous risk of these lifestyle associated diseases. We [in the US] focus on individuals and that has shown to have limited efficacy and now it's probably time for us to focus on larger issues.

Former New York City Mayor Michael Bloomberg has been a leader in this initiative to protect children from a lifetime of obesity related chronic diseases. Education for adults and children is key and government should do everything possible to assure that we are all getting the facts about the risks of overweight and obesity and what we have to do to protect ourselves and our families. University of Memphis' James Gurney, Ph.D. says that overweight and obesity:

...is a very, very strong cultural issue that has proven to be rather intractable and it will have to be a multidimensional approach and is not going to be easily solved. If we are going to get a handle on this from a societal standpoint, the government will have to be heavily involved. If we think we are going to solve this problem one by one, then I think we are going to be very disappointed in the long run...There are very strong financial incentives across many, many industries that are going to be very resistant toward allowing a cohesive message that's homogeneous and targeted to kids.

Starting with children is especially important since the best way to maintain a normal weight is to not get overweight or obese to begin with. Losing weight is much harder than not becoming over-weight or obese. Lynn Panton, Ph.D., Associate Professor at Florida State University explains:

> We have to start young because it's very difficult once you're older, and you have these bad habits. That's not to say you can't change because you can but it's a lot easier to start with your children and educate them and try to get them to exercise. It's a lot easier to keep the weight off when you're young than when you're older. We have to educate our children and help them to be active as they get older and teach them about the proper food choices. It is very difficult once you're older to change those behaviors.

University of Illinois' John Erdman, Ph.D. points out that:

> Obesity and overweight starts at a very young age and it's very difficult to get off of that…so early prevention of child-hood obesity is going to be very critical for the next genera-tion…my personal feeling is that getting to the very young children is the way to go…

Robert Amato, D.O., Chief of the Division of Oncology at Memorial Hermann Cancer Center says:

> With obesity, where we can impact the most is with children. They are still young. Their minds are still open and they have not gone through the pitfalls we have as adults. It's not just educating them at school, it's also educating their parents.

The University of Kentucky's Mark Dignan, Ph.D. notes that with the obesity issue:

> One of the areas where we really need to intervene is in schools because when we have school policies that don't

address obesity in children, we are really missing an opportunity here to have people get off on the right foot...

Given the challenges, can we be successful at getting control of
the obesity epidemic in the United States? Probably, but it's going
to take an all-out effort similar to one required to get the smoking
rates way down in the US. Harvard University's Walter Willet, M.D.,
Dr. P.H. says he believes we do need an all-out war against obesity:

> We need to pull out as many stops as we can including eco-
> nomics and working on prevention and helping people who
> are already seriously overweight...I don't think we should
> be totally discouraged by looking at the studies of people
> regaining weight because it's very similar to what we saw in
> smoking. Smoking is addictive and very hard to break and
> the best interventions only run about 10 or 12% success rate
> for smoking cessation by the end of the year but when peo-
> ple repeatedly keep trying and keep working on it, we have
> dropped smoking rates in men from about 60% to less than
> 20% over 40 years, it took us a long time... We shouldn't
> forget that there are a lot of people who have incorporated
> healthy eating and physical activity into their lives and are
> controlling their weight and without that it would be even
> much worse than it is today...If we were really serious about
> it, we can get back a long ways. In some ways it's more
> complicated and challenging than reversing the tobacco
> epidemic. I don't really see any reason why it's not possible
> to have a very major change but it will probably require a
> generation or two to achieve that.

University of Colorado's Tim Byers, M.D., M.P.H. adds:

> I am not very fatalistic about this whole issue because I think
> if you look at the obesity trends worldwide there are sev-
> eral countries that have begun to turn around the obesity

epidemic in Europe, Scandinavia. Here in the US, the rate of obesity increase has flattened off. Over the last decade we are not increasing like we were and if you look at the US, there are these big social class disparities where people who are at higher SES levels, richer people, are less obese than people who are lower SES, poorer people - that all gives me hope that we can actually and will turn around the obesity epidemic. We are not all going to get skinny again but I think we are going to begin to turn around the obesity epidemic here. I think the social denormalization that's worked for tobacco will probably work for things like huge soft drinks, oversized portions of fatty foods in restaurants and things like that. If you go to a high class restaurant now, you don't get a gob of food on your plate but rather a small serving. I think those are indicators that we are going to turn around the way we look at food.

To be successful on this issue, communities will have to be involved by providing playgrounds and other facilities where children can be physically active as well as walking paths for adults and encourage grocery stores to carry healthy foods. Parents will need to change their own bad eating behaviors and be good role models for their children. Gordon Saxe, M.D., Ph.D., Director for the Center for Integrative Medicine at University of California, San Diego says there is more awareness on the part of parents:

> Kids are an incredibly important population...there's nothing more important than what happens early in life as we are setting the stage for a lifetime of habits. I am optimistic that can occur because I've seen a lot of interest and growing interest among parents. They recognize that there is, in the American food supply, a problem and the way our sedentary lifestyle happens, and I think there is a growing awareness and the need for their kids to get onto healthy things early.

Exercise and Physical Activity

Lack of exercise and physical activity is a risk factor for cancer as well as heart disease. While some health conscious people consistently exercise, most do not. University of Houston's Tracey Ledoux, Ph.D. says, "Eating and not exercising are the norm in our society....". As noted earlier, throughout most of human existence, people were physically active and our bodies evolved requiring certain amounts of physical activity to be healthy. What do experts say about lack of exercise and cancer risk? Anthony Shield, M.D., Associate Director of the Barbara Ann Karmanos Cancer Institute at Wayne State University says, "Increasing exercise decreases cancer risk." Robert Hiatt M.D., Ph.D., Chair, Department of Epidemiology at the University of California, San Francisco points out that, "Physical activity has been found to reduce the consequences of cancer and may reduce the onset of cancer or the occurrence of cancer." Lynn Panton, Ph.D., Associate Professor at Florida State University says, "Exercise is so important in helping to prevent all kinds of chronic diseases including breast cancer and prostate cancer." University of California, Davis' Marc Schenker, M.D., M.P.H. notes that, "Lack of physical inactivity is associated with increased cancer risk." University of Arizona's Peter Lance, M.D. says, "Lead a generally healthy lifestyle. Increasingly, obesity and factors that go with obesity are the lack of physical activity and exercise over a lifetime, they are very important risk factors for not just cancer but most of the common chronic diseases." Louisiana State University's Edward Trapido, Ph.D. adds, "Make sure you get a reasonable amount of exercise because that has been associated with decreased risk of colon cancer for example." John Vena, Ph.D., Professor of Epidemiology at the Medical University of South Carolina says, "Exercise and increased physical activity has been shown to reduce risks for a number of cancers."

Unfortunately, however, our busy, sedentary lifestyle in the US and throughout the developed world has been working against us.

Many people have office jobs and too many come home at night after work and spend hours sitting in front of the television and in more recent years, the computer. Melinda Irwin, Ph.D., Co-Director of the Cancer Prevention and Control Program at Yale University explains:

> Over the last 10 years, the biggest change in the United States has been with people's leisure time, what they do outside of work? The biggest change has been technological advances...1995 is when people regularly got on the computer and they're on it all the time whether it's Facebook or Twitter or just Googling stuff. That's how they're spending their leisure time...which could lead to a half a pound of weight gain per week or 6 pounds per year...20 or 30 years ago we did not have as much obesity...because we have completely changed our lifestyle. We are way more sedentary than we have ever been before...and why don't people lose weight? It's more exciting to go on the computer and Google and go on Facebook. You have these distractions that for most people are more enjoyable than going out and exercising. When people only have one or two hours of leisure time per day, how are they choosing to use it.

John Pierce, Ph.D., Professor of Family and Preventative Medicine and Co-Leader of the Cancer Prevention Program at the Moores Cancer Center at the University of California, San Diego adds, "If you have a predilection toward obesity and you give up exercise, then you're going to be in trouble...". Christine Curran, Ph.D., Assistant Professor of Biology at Northern Kentucky University points out that in addition:

> The types of jobs we have today have changed dramatically. My dad's generation was working, the generation before people were out on the farms, the jobs tended to be more physically active and not sitting in front of computers...which

doesn't involve a whole lot of calorie burning...If we want to go somewhere, we get in the car. 'I am not going to get on a bike, I am not going to walk' [is the norm for most]...

It is important to understand that health experts recommend exercise <u>and</u> physical activity. Exercise is a regular planned program of physical activity such as walking, jogging, swimming, biking and resistance exercise such as weight lifting. The American Heart Association and others recommend at least 30 minutes of moderate exercise like walking almost every day to meet the minimum guidelines of 150 minutes per week. Alternatively, a minimum or 75 minutes per week (i.e., 15 minutes per day) of vigorous exercise like jogging or swimming which is also a great form of exercise. Paul Walker, M.D., Director of Oncology at the Brady School of Medicine at East Carolina University says:

> The two things that make a difference, one is aerobic exercise and for anybody obese that is clearly walking. You are not training for a marathon, you are not out to walk 5 miles the first day, do what you can do and if you need to throw in some rest days, you aim for five days a week, 30 minutes of walking...and some muscle strengthening exercises like resistance bands or light weightlifting with more frequent repetitions in which the resistance will stimulate an anti-inflammatory process in the body which is the whole key and how it impacts cancer [prevention].

Vigorous aerobic exercise can also improve mental health in addition to improving your physical health and reducing cancer risk. One recent study that compared walking to jogging concluded that to achieve the maximum health benefits, the distance traveled matters more than which of those two forms of exercise was used. If you have a chronic medical condition, consult with your primary care physician prior to starting your exercise program. In addition to aerobic exercise, the American Heart Association emphasizes muscle strengthening exercises at least twice per week using as many muscle groups as possible. To maximize strength development, a resistance (weight) should be used that allows 8 to 10 repetitions producing muscle fatigue. Muscle strengthening activities include a progressive weight training program, weight-bearing calisthenics, stair climbing, or similar resistance exercises that use the major muscle groups. For example, you might consider weight lifting once per week for the upper body - arms, neck, back, abdomen and then once per week for the lower body doing a variety of leg and lower back exercises.

Studies have demonstrated that people also need physical activity throughout the day to reduce cancer risk further which is challenging due to our sedentary lifestyle but can be done with thoughtful, conscious effort. Moffit Cancer Center's Thomas Sellers, Ph.D., M.P.H. says, "Physical activity does not have to mean going to the gym for intense aerobic activity although that's good. Being active, walking rather than driving around for an hour to park in the front row, park in the back and walk there. Standing rather than sitting helps burn calories." Workplaces and universities can also help to encourage physical activity during the day as can the use of social support such as walking with a "buddy". University of North Carolina, Chapel Hill's Kurt Ribisl, Ph.D. explains:

> One of the things I'm a big fan of is using behavioral economics to help people...change health behaviors...get a 'buddy' - social support is a key thing...At our School of Public Health they designed a stair case to be really attractive...and that encouraged people to walk...putting art and music in there is causing lots more people to use the stairwell.

Like most changes to improve health and reduce risk of cancer and other chronic diseases, staying with an exercise program can be challenging. Louisiana State University's Melinda Sothern, Ph.D. says:

I, as an exercise physiologist, that's where I tend to want to push people more toward the physical side of it only because it is the side that is mostly ignored and it is the side that individuals really have a difficult time changing. It is very difficult for them, cognitively, behaviorally, physically - to make that decision to become more physically active for long enough to have what we call the 'training effect' which is really what you want and what really prevents these diseases to begin with. Cancer, being an inflammatory condition, exercise training lowers oxidative stress, lowers free radical activity that promotes cancer.

Many people have busy lifestyles and other issues in their lives that they use as an excuse not to exercise. Yale University's Melinda Irwin, Ph.D. explains:

When I recruit patients for my [weight loss] research studies, people will say, 'I really need this but I don't want to do it right now.' Either they are too busy or they are not really wanting to eat healthier or exercise even though they know they should. They're just like, 'Oh, got other things on my plate'...maybe they are trying to quit smoking; maybe they have some financial issues going on; maybe they've got work issues and right now they really can't deal with it.

Of course, these types of everyday problems are quite common in real life and people need to avoid dealing with stress in self-destructive ways and instead find healthy alternatives to deal with life's problems. Dr. Sothern explains, "Stress contributes to disease and it's very important to keep your stress down with activities like physical activity, meditation, yoga and things like that. The worst thing you can do is deal with stress in destructive ways such as turning to alcohol, cigarettes, and over-eating." People who find a way to start exercising often discover that it reduces stress, improves clarity of thinking and mental health which can help them deal more effectively with their problems. Carlos Crespo, Ph.D., Professor of Community Health at Portland State University notes, "If you ask people who exercise regularly, most of them are doing it as a stress reliever. It's just a habit, they feel better when they exercise."

When starting an exercise program, it is better to start slow and implement a moderate program of exercise which is more sustainable in the long term. Later, you always have the option of gradually increasing the length of the exercise program. Pebbles Fagan, Ph.D., M.P.H., Associate Professor of Prevention and Control at the University of Hawaii Cancer Center says, "We recommend that people be physically active at a moderate or intense level for at least 30 minutes a day every day...walking, gardening, running, swimming. Going from 30 minutes a day to an hour a day is not a far reach for many people." For those who are unable or unwilling to get a regular exercise program going, increased physical activity can help. Wendy Pogezelski, Ph.D., Professor of Chemistry at State University of New York Geneseo, explains:

> I think people have this idea that exercise means going to the gym and really that's not playing out...We all need more movement throughout the entire day...We really have to be working our muscles...Certainly going to the gym is beneficial...but really if people increase their movement throughout the day it really helps.

There are some people, because of their current physical condition, including medical issues, that may face some additional obstacles but those can be overcome with a little creativity and effort. John Spangler, M.D., M.S., a Family Medicine physician at Wake Forest Baptist Medical Center, says some patients "...who have osteoarthritis of the knee, etc. - finding some way they can get themselves moving to some extent whether it's using their upper body, lifting weights, doing arm exercises, or walking around the house or a treadmill at home - getting patients moving is important...".

Exercise should not be your sole weight loss strategy as it must be combined with a nutritious well-balanced diet to be successful. Lynn Panton, Ph.D., Associate Professor at Florida State University says, "Exercise alone will not fix the problem if you are going to eat out of control." Remember, the Journal of Clinical Diabetes study above that noted the characteristics of people who successfully maintain weight loss – among those characteristics were regular exercise and a healthy diet. Ohio State University's Peter Shields, M.D., adds, "Eat a well-balanced diet…and exercise to maintain a healthy weight." Yale Cancer Center's Maura Harrigan, M.S., R.D. reminds us that, "Achieving and maintaining a healthy weight [is accomplished through a] combination of healthy eating and physical activity - they go hand-in-hand."

6

Environmental Chemicals

Environmental synthetic chemicals are becoming an ever-increasing cancer risk due to the tens of thousands of untested chemicals in our environment in the United States. Synthetic chemicals are those that are manmade as opposed to naturally occurring chemicals found in nature. Throughout this chapter, we will use the term "environmental chemicals" or "chemicals" to mean manmade chemicals and not keep repeating the term "synthetic".

As noted earlier in the brief review of evolution and cancer, we know that the environment in which humans evolved is far different than the one we live in today and our bodies are not catching up to the relatively rapid changes from the industrial revolution over the last couple of hundred years and the chemical revolution in recent decades. Charnita Zeigler-Johnson, Ph.D., M.P.H., Professor of Cancer Epidemiology at Thomas Jefferson University says, "I do believe we are living in a world now where we are exposed to so many more potential carcinogens than in the past." The National Cancer Institute states that being exposed to chemicals and other substances in the environment has been linked to some cancers. As noted earlier, the President's Cancer Panel report in 2009 expressed serious concern explaining, "With nearly 80,000 chemicals on the market in the United States, many of which are used by millions of Americans in their daily lives and are un or understudied and largely unregulated, exposure to potential environmental carcinogens is widespread." It was also noted in an earlier chapter that the the

American Academy of Pediatrics says that babies in America are born "pre-polluted", getting many of these chemicals from their mothers before they are even born and recently, the International Agency for Cancer Research, the organization that the world looks to evaluate potentially carcinogenic substances, declared air pollution to be a "known carcinogen".

We also ingest many synthetic chemical substances through our food and water, the latter which is supposed to help remove toxins from our cells not add them. As mentioned earlier, in an exhaustive review of drinking water in the United States, the New York Times concluded that many contaminants in our drinking water are not monitored by the EPA noting that, "At least 62 million Americans have been exposed since 2004 to drinking water that did not meet at least one commonly used government health guideline intended to help protect people from cancer...". The observation that babies in America are born "pre-polluted" comes at a time when childhood cancers are increasing in the US. Old Dominion University's Richard Heller, Ph.D. says while although older people generally have a higher cancer risk, "Unfortunately, younger and younger people are getting cancer which is really depressing." Wayne Sanderson, Ph.D., Professor and Chair of Epidemiology at the University of Kentucky says, "We are exposed to a tremendous number of chemicals. Every two years, the National Toxicology Program puts out their report on carcinogens. There is evidence that we are exposed to a lot of carcinogens - a high number of them...".

It is also interesting that while most of the cancer risks presented in this book are widely accepted among cancer experts, there are some differences of opinion over how much danger environmental chemicals pose. Yet, there seems to be unanimity among cancer experts that smoking is the number one cause of cancer and number one cause of preventable death in United States and throughout the world and what is smoking if not the release of chemicals into the smoker produced from the burning and inhaling of tobacco smoke, with a number of those chemicals being carcinogenic. According to the National Cancer Institute, "Among the 250 known harmful chemicals in tobacco smoke, at least 69 can cause cancer."

Time after time we find out that some of these environmental chemical substances are harmful long after many millions of Americans have been exposed to them. For example, the US government used to put cigarettes in the rations of American soldiers during World War I. Companies used to put asbestos, what now a known carcinogen, in children's' schools. Manufacturers put lead in gasoline and paint until we learned of its harmful health effects. As noted earlier, air pollution was recently declared to be a carcinogen and yet we have been spewing massive amounts of toxic chemicals into the air we breathe for decades. Jia-Sheng Wang, M.D., Ph.D., Professor and Head of Environmental Health Sciences at the University of Georgia says, "You think there is no toxicity and no carcinogenicity in a lot of chemicals but later on you find out, it's not true."

In addition, we used to spray the pesticide, DDT, over much of our produce which serves as a good example of the problems that environmental chemicals can pose. Michael Skinner, Ph.D., Professor of Biochemistry at Washington State University explains, "In the 1950s, for 10 years, the entire North American population was exposed to DDT extensively - we fogged cities and towns, sprayed it on every crop we had. DDT was heavily used for 10 years until we realized there was a problem and then we stopped." Anna Jeng, Ph.D., Associate Professor and Director of the School of Community and Environmental Health at Old Dominion University says that all these years later, DDT is still a problem noting:

> DDT was banned in the 1970s...but it takes a long time to break down...and was found not long ago in the Mississippi River and the Gulf Coast...and in the soil...When it gets in the body even in small concentrations, it accumulates in your

fat tissue and will stay there for a long time - 30 or 40 years, enough to do bad things to your body.

Anthony Shield, M.D., Associate Director of the Barbara Ann Karmanos Cancer Institute at Wayne State University concurs saying:

> Limiting our chemical exposure is certainly a reasonable idea and goal...We have done studies here, for instance, with DDT which was subsequently banned as a pesticide but we have data from patients with pancreatic cancer showing that they had increased levels decades after their exposure. DDT is something that dissolves in the fat in our body and really stays there for many, many years.

This is not implying that all synthetic chemicals are harmful but we should have learned by now that what we don't know can kill us. Matthew Gage, Ph.D., Professor of Chemistry and Biochemistry at Northern Arizona University says, "Look at Madame Curie. Here is someone who was one of the first people to study radiation and it killed her because she didn't know what she was getting exposed to... I think the Precautionary Principle is valuable." University of Minnesota's Robert Turesky, Ph.D. adds, "We are exposed to various mutagenic, genotoxic, potentially carcinogenic chemicals in our diet, in our environment every single day...That chemicals are safe until proven unsafe, that seems to me to be potentially problematic in its orientation."

It is worth repeating the earlier quote by Michael Gurven, Ph.D., an Evolutionary Anthropologist from the University of California, Santa Barbara who noted that, "There are tons of exposures we would have not had in the past...Anything that has changed dramatically in the past, let's say, 50 years certainly our ability to adapt genetically is 'zero'." That statement is particularly relevant in this discussion of environmental synthetic chemicals given that most of the 80,000 chemicals referenced in the President's Cancer Panel report were introduced in just the last 50 years.

The Great Chemical Divide

Why is there a difference of opinion among some cancer experts as to the amount of cancer risk these environmental synthetic chemicals pose? In part, some feel that we have not seen enough increase in the incidence rates of cancers commensurate with all of the chemicals introduced in recent decades or that perceived increases of some cancers might just be that we are detecting cancers better with improved technology. Christine Curran, Ph.D., Assistant Professor of Biology at Northern Kentucky University explains the dilemma:

> Thyroid cancers are on the rise and there doesn't seem to be a good understanding as to why although some people say we have gotten better at finding them, that it's not a true increase but just an increase in the identification as we have gotten more sophisticated on how we do our screening.

Others believe that we are seeing sufficient evidence of real increases in certain cancers. Dean Hosgood, Ph.D., M.P.H., at Albert Einstein College of Medicine asks:

> What is leading to this increase? As we are looking for clues, we can look at genetic, environment and lifestyle factors - there are tremendous efforts ongoing to try to find out some of those clues and we are doing studies...While we are able to detect cancers better than we had before, that is not the cause of the increase, people believe there is a true increase in cancers rates such as thyroid and lymphomas.

Tongzhang Zheng, D.Sc., Professor of Epidemiology at the Yale School of Medicine and Consultant to the World Health Organization agrees that there are real and significant increases in a number of cancers explaining, "There are many, many cancers increasing...Liver cancer is increasing, thyroid cancer is increasing, Hodgkin's disease particularly among younger people is increasing...Testicular cancer has been increasing, non-Hodgkin's lymphoma has been increasing, pancreatic cancer is increasing."

There are some cancer experts, however, who would like to see more evidence of the widespread potential effects of chemicals on cancer such as University of Colorado's Tim Byers, M.D., M.P.H. who says:

> The best evidence that we have from studies is that really there are not big environmental causes of cancer such as pesticides and herbicides and food tolerance and things like that... Those same compounds when given in high doses can be carcinogenic but in very, very low, diluted out doses - those are detoxified [in our bodies] by the same mechanisms that detoxify naturally occurring carcinogens in our foods...We will find some evidence of some environmental chemicals that even at low doses cause cancer but is it likely that environmental contaminants are explaining an appreciable part of cancer burden here in the US - I don't think so.

Thomas Kensler, Ph.D., Professor of Cancer Pharmacology and Cancer Prevention, at the University of Pittsburgh adds:

> We haven't seen over the last few decades, with the exception of lung cancer and cigarette smoking, we have not seen huge changes in [cancer] rates. In some cases they are going down and in other cases they are going up but there have not been these precipitous swings which would suggest we've introduce something into the environment or something has changed dramatically in risk that a decade or two

later is following it...That's not to say that we haven't got products where we are going to look back and say 'That was a mistake' - for sure we have chemicals in production that we are going to wish we didn't have.

However, others like Laura Vanderberg, Ph.D., Professor of Environmental Health at University of Massachusetts School of Public Health Sciences believes there is sufficient evidence that environmental synthetic chemicals are indeed a significant problem:

> Rates of certain cancers have increased in ways that we cannot explain...To use breast cancer as an example, in the 1940s, a woman's risk of getting breast cancer was one in 22. Today, it's somewhere around one in eight. That's the difference between my grandmother's generation and my generation. The number of genetic changes between grandma and me are so few that they cannot explain this increase in risk. What can explain it is this boom in the production of chemicals. Largely, these are chemicals we don't know anything about. The chemicals that we do know about, high production chemicals that have been studied more extensively, there is cause for concern.

Albert Cunningham, Ph.D., Associate Professor of Public Health at the University of Louisville adds, "Benzene is a classic example because it is a known carcinogen and we go out and get ourselves exposed to benzene every time we pump gasoline...". The National Institute of Environmental Health's Linda Birnbaum, Ph.D. agrees with the President's Cancer Panel and American Academy of Pediatrics quotes above describing the concern about chemicals in our environment saying, "I don't think they are overstating the situation. We do know that if you monitor what is in newborn babies, they have many, many different environmental synthetic chemicals that are present in their bodies..."

Even chemicals used ostensibly for health reasons can sometimes turn out to actually cause cancer. Wichita State University's William Hendry, Ph.D. says:

> There is clear evidence that there are agents that have been proven to lead to cancer as well as endocrine disruption...For example, a chemical called DES was used from the 1940s until the 1970s because they thought it would prevent miscarriages and it turned out to be a result of misinterpretation of some studies and not only did it not prevent miscarriages but maybe even enhanced them but more importantly it caused the placenta to be exposed and developing fetuses to this very, very strong estrogen that caused rare forms of uterine cancer and also a disruption of the reproductive tract. Over 2 million fetuses in the United States were exposed to that so there is actually support group for what's called 'DES Daughters and Sons'...

Dartmouth Medical School's Angeline Andrew, Ph.D. points out that:

> There is new information in recent years that the proportion of cancers that can be attributed to environmental exposures may be higher than previously thought...From that perspective, I think that increases our responsibility and our ability to prevent cancers.

Yale School of Medicine's Tongzhang Zheng, D.Sc. says, "I fully agree" with the President Cancer Panel statement and adds:

> Thyroid cancer is increasing very rapidly in the United States. What's the reason? It is very possible that it is due to the chemicals... We have not fully recognized how these 80,000 chemicals affect us...and how they are metabolized in our bodies and how they interact with our genetic makeup...

These chemicals that enter our body may form new chemicals which may be more harmful than their original form... chemicals are part of the modern world we enjoy...but we should avoid as much unnecessary exposure as we can.

Traditional thinking has been that environmental exposures to synthetic chemicals causes a relatively small percentage of cancers. Louisiana State University's Edward Trapido, Ph.D. explains:

There are a lot of chemicals associated with cancer and increased risk but in terms of the general population exposures as a percentage of all cancer deaths attributable to chemicals, it's on the relatively low side...There have only been a few evaluations that have tried to pin down the proportion of cancer deaths attributable to certain factors... Whether it's 3%, or 5%, or 8%, is not really the big issue. The big issue is if that it's not 3% but 30%, that would be a big deal...I'm not sure if 3% is the right answer, and it might be 5% and it might be 8% but it's not 30%. We don't have a lot of confidence in a very specific number, but we know whether something is likely to be a major cause of cancer death or a small cause of cancer death and maybe this will change but my suspicion is that it will be a while before we go from 3% to 20%. The people who have done these studies are very qualified epidemiologists and other researchers.

On the other hand, some think that the percentage of cancers caused by environmental chemicals is higher than traditionally thought. Rashmi Kaul, Ph.D., Associate Professor of Immunology at Oklahoma State University Center explains:

I totally believe that these chemicals can directly affect our immune responses because immune cells have receptors which can be affected by these chemicals and then our immune responses will not act in a way that can effectively attack cancer cells. As an immunologist, I know that the immune system is constantly monitoring for these cancer cells and constantly keeping them in check but if the immune system gets affected by the chemicals, you can see the increase in auto-immune diseases, in which your immune system is attacking its own cells - it is getting misled by these chemicals, and some autoimmune diseases lead to cancer. All of these immune disorders are leading either into autoimmune diseases or cancer...I think we are underestimating the percentage of cancers that are caused by chemicals which I believe is definitely about 10% and may cause between 20% and 30% of all cancers, or even more, whether they are diagnosed or undiagnosed, if you include both direct and indirect effects because chemicals affect immune cells which then are not able to clear some of the infections which can lead to more cancers.

Old Dominion University's Anna Jeng, Ph.D. adds, "Estimates that 5% of cancers are caused by environmental exposure underestimate, for example, toxins that come from our air, water, plastic bottles on a daily basis...".

Given that 580,000 American will die of cancer in 2014, whether the percentage of cancer deaths caused by environmental chemicals is 3%, 5%,10%, 20% or higher - it is too high if avoiding these chemicals by using by using the Precautionary Principle can help save many of those lives. Dale Shepard, M.D., Ph.D., a medical oncologist with the Cleveland Clinic asks, "Is it likely that there are a lot of environmental factors that we don't understand - absolutely...and the tragic thing is that we do know that so many of them do cause cancer and we don't do enough about it." University of Arizona's Peter Lance, M.D. says, "There are people who banged on about something and were told they were wrong for 10, 20 or 30 years then, 'Okay, by the way, tobacco is indeed harmful'...I think one always has to be careful of not missing something that's sitting right under your nose." On the other hand, Walter Willet, M.D., Dr. P.H., Professor of Epidemiology and Nutrition and Chair of the Department of Nutrition at the Harvard School of Public Health reminds us, "I am a precautionary person too but it's important to put what you're being precautious about in balance and not forget about the bigger, very solid, very well substantiated very powerful factors like smoking and obesity." Hopefully, Americans are resourceful enough to focus on all of these serious threats to their health and to the health of their families.

General Agreement on the Use of the Precautionary Principle for Environmental Chemicals

Even though there may be some differences on the extent of the cancer threat from environmental chemicals which will likely become clearer with more data as the years go on, there is widespread agreement that the vast majority of these chemicals have not been tested adequately for human safety and therefore considerable support for the use of what cancer experts refer to as the "Precautionary Principle". The Precautionary Principle is a strategy to cope with possible risks where scientific understanding is not yet complete. One dictionary defines it as, "The precept that an action should not be taken if the consequences are uncertain or potentially dangerous". It is often applied to public policy but also applies to individuals to reduce risks in their own lives and in those of their families. Erin Eaton, Ph.D., Associate Professor of Biology at Francis Marion University summarizes the principle simply explaining, "I totally agree with the Precautionary Principle...It's better to be safe than sorry." This is pretty much what our mothers taught us. In the case of environmental synthetic chemicals, the Precautionary Principle means avoiding untested chemicals to the extent possible. Robert Hiatt M.D., Ph.D., Chair, Department of Epidemiology at the University of California, San Francisco explains, "The Precautionary Principle is, even if you're not sure about the danger of some of these environmental exposures, why not just not expose myself to them until there is better information."

Even cancer experts who are not convinced that the risks of environmental chemicals is substantial, often agree with the use of the Precautionary Principle including the two cancer experts quoted above, Drs. Kensler and Byers. University of Pittsburgh's Dr. Kensler explains, "There is a movement toward the Precautionary Principle to try to avoid potential exposures even if we really don't have the risk dynamics fully defined...As a toxicologist I argue for the Precautionary Principle of more information in advance as a laudable goal and approach." In a discussion around the chemicals, BPAs and Phthalates, and their health risks, Dr. Byers advised, "If you have the option to avoid it, just go ahead and avoid it." A third cancer expert who shares those views, UC San Diego's John Pierce, Ph.D. says, "The environmental causes of cancer are much smaller than what advocates claim but people should use the Precautionary Principle, absolutely."

Bill Fields, Ph.D., M.S., Professor of Epidemiology at the University of Iowa says of the President's Cancer Panel quote above, "I think that's right on target." He adds that the use of the Precautionary Principle "is a perfectly logical and reasonable approach...We are being exposed to so many chemicals that have never been tested and weren't even on the market 10 years ago, anything you can do that's reasonable to try to reduce risk exposure to chemicals is really helpful...". Moffit Cancer Center's Thomas Sellers, Ph.D., M.P.H. adds, "Absolutely, the Precautionary Principle is a good idea. It is a good idea to avoid known exposure whenever possible...It doesn't hurt to do whatever we can to lower our risk."

There is especially concern around some ubiquitous chemicals in everyday use including PCBs and phthalates that are in billions of plastic bottles, cans containing beverage and food and plastic bags used in the home. University of California, Davis' Marc Schenker,

M.D., M.P.H. illustrates the use of the Precautionary Principle with BPAs in plastics explaining:

> BPAs...is a reactive chemical but most importantly it's not necessary. It is purely a commercial creation that we don't need so those are the cases where I say, yes, let's get rid of it...Even if we haven't established it as a human carcinogen. We don't need it. Some people call that the Precautionary Principle. While it's not an established carcinogen, it's certainly not good for you and maybe it's bad in ways we don't know and we can do away with it.

Brown University's Karl Kelsey, M.D., M.P.H. says, "I do think it makes more sense to apply the Precautionary Principle where it's possible to apply it reasonably." Jay Thomas Sutliffe, Ph.D., Associate Professor of Public Health at Northern Arizona University adds, "We are definitely in a toxic environment...We should avoid as much of it as possible...I am a huge proponent of, in the immediate, at looking at how I could change my environment at work, my office, how can I do it at home, what I put in my body - I am big on individual responsibility."

Individuals and Families: Implementing the Precautionary Principle in Your Day-to-Day Life

Drink Filtered or Distilled Water

Specifically, what actions should individuals and their families take to implement the Precautionary Principle in their own lives when it comes to environmental chemicals? A good starting point is to think about how these chemicals get into our bodies – from what we eat, drink, and breathe as well as through our skin. A good starting point is with drinking water since the body is comprised of 60% water for the average adult and health experts recommend that we drink eight glasses of water a day for optimal health. Moreover, it has long been known that clean drinking water is important to human health. While it is often thought that America's drinking water is safe, people may want to rethink that assumption. It is true that the quality of our drinking water is better than many countries in the world, but that does not mean that it is truly safe and it varies widely by community. There are many chemicals in our drinking water that have never even been tested for human safety. The *New York Times* conducted an exhaustive review of the US water supply that uncovered troubling information and published an extensive article that concluded in part:

> Only 91 contaminants are regulated under the safe drinking water act...government and independent scientists...identified hundreds associated with the risks of cancer and other diseases in small concentrations in drinking water...but not one chemical has been added to the list of those regulated by the Safe Drinking Water Act since 2000...Government scientists now generally agree that many chemicals commonly found in drinking water pose serious risks even at low concentrations...Independent studies in such journals as: Reviews of Environmental Contamination and Toxicology; Environmental Health Perspectives; American Journal of Public Health; Archives of Environmental and Occupational Health; and, reports published by the National Academy of Sciences suggested millions of Americans become sick each year from drinking contaminated water, with maladies from upset stomachs to cancer and birth defects...EPA administrator Lisa Jackson said, 'Since chemicals are ubiquitous in our economy, our environment...we need better authority so we can assure the public that any unacceptable risks have been eliminated...but under existing law, we cannot give that assurance.'...Linda Birnbaum who is the Director of the National Institute of Environmental Health Science said, 'These chemicals accumulate in body tissue and affect developmental and hormonal systems in ways we don't

understand. There's growing evidence that numerous chemicals are more dangerous than previously thought, but the EPA is still going to give them a clean bill of health'.

University of Iowa's Bill Fields, Ph.D., M.S. points out that, "Not all potential exposures are monitored in our water systems." University of Pittsburgh's Thomas Kensler, Ph.D. says that most municipal water supplies in the US are pretty good and do a good job at neutralizing biological organisms that were a cause of infectious diseases in the past. However, he adds:

> Is the water supply in the United States uniformly pristine? No, certainly not. We have our brown fields and industrial legacies, contaminated aquifers in different areas and smaller municipalities that really can't afford to screen for those sorts of things which are more uncertain particularly if they are located near old industrial sites.

Old Dominion University's Anna Jeng, Ph.D. says, "Our drinking water systems are not designed to remove many toxic compounds. Our water treatment systems basically just remove some contaminants…". Dragos Albinescu, Ph.D., Associate Professor of Chemistry at Northeastern State University adds:

> Drinking water is not tested for everything that it contains. There are not regulations to protect you from everything in your drinking water…My concern is what I see in my sink when water evaporates and the sink is covered with stains, spots which look horrible to me…We don't know what's in our drinking water…

Brown University's Dr. Kelsey adds, "The regulatory arena around water and water contaminations certainly has problems. I think public water supplies should be better regulated and certainly better monitored." Georgetown University's Laura Anderko,

Ph.D., R.N. adds that one should be, "...very critical in your thinking about what you purchase, what you eat, what you drink. Water filters can take out a lot of chemicals and harmful agents from your water - it's not 100% clean but it's cleaner than anything you will get from your tap...". Robert Hiatt M.D., Ph.D., Chair, Department of Epidemiology at the University of California, San Francisco recommends, "...reducing environmental exposure to environmental carcinogens that we know exist not only in polluted air and water...". Washington State University's Michael Skinner, Ph.D. says what he would advise any prospective mother is to, "Be very cautious about your water source...Your biggest contamination to a degree is your water source...The first thing for the average person is to not drink tap water, you have to drink purified water, particularly if you are pregnant." Susan Arnold, M.D., Associate Professor of Medical Oncology and Radiation Medicine at the Markey Cancer Center and the University of Kentucky says, "No one in eastern Kentucky drinks their tap water [they use a lot of well water]. They already know because they have seen life after life after life taken to cancer and other diseases."

Chemicals get into our water supply from a variety of sources including chemicals used as fertilizers and pesticides that get into ground water tables. Dean Hosgood, Ph.D., M.P.H., at Albert Einstein College of Medicine says, "When it comes to the US...we do know the drinking water is coming from our groundwater tables where a lot of environmental exposures have leached into the groundwater...". Barbara McCahan, Ph.D., Professor of Health and Physical Education at Plymouth State University adds that, "In the process of fracking, I have seen the devastation to the landscape that is happening...They are leaving huge pools of fluid that once were water and now fully contaminated with hydrocarbon type chemicals." University of Massachusetts' Laura Vanderberg, Ph.D. adds, "Right now we are seeing this play out in West Virginia with the terrible leak at a coal production plant. A chemical that was released into the waterways there, there's almost nothing known about that chemical." Laura Anderko, Ph.D., R.N. says, "The pharmaceuticals in our water is huge. The fact that people are on chemotherapeutic agents and they go to the bathroom and those agents are radioactive and end up in our water supply."

Occasionally, in addition to synthetic chemicals, naturally occurring substances can also appear in drinking water that cause health problems such as arsenic which has been classified by the EPA as a human carcinogen. It is an odorless and tasteless semi-metal which can enter water from natural deposits in the earth and air from natural processes such as volcanoes but also from industrial processes – it is used as a wood preservative but also in paints, dyes, metals, drugs and soaps. The National Resources Defense Council estimates that between 34 and 56 million Americans in the 25 states that report arsenic levels to the EPA were drinking tap water from systems containing average levels of arsenic that posed unacceptable cancer risks. The National Academy of Sciences studies have concluded that arsenic in drinking water causes cancer, including bladder and lung cancer. Robert Goyer, chair of the committee who wrote the Academy report said, "Even low concentrations of arsenic in drinking water appear to be associated with a higher incidence of cancer."

What steps should people take to deal with toxins in our drinking water? Angeline Andrew, Ph.D., a Molecular Epidemiologist and Assistant Professor of Community and Family Medicine at the Geisel School of Medicine at Dartmouth Medical School says, "I would recommend people test their water... Getting your water tested and knowing what's in there is important." Whether you test your water or not, people would be well advised to switch from drinking tap water to using steam distilled or filtered water. Northern Arizona University's Matthew Gage, Ph.D. explains:

> Water quality is a big issue. The more you do to purify your water, the healthier you are going to be. Distilling it or using

filters, there's a lot of things you can do to try and take out a lot of the factors that are in the water. Distilling it may be the best way to go although there may still be just a little residual that has the same boiling point as water but you are certainly going to clean out a lot of things.

In fact, a number of cancer experts take steps in their personal lives to use filtered or distilled water including John Vena, Ph.D., Professor of Epidemiology at the Medical University of South Carolina who says, "In my own house, for cooking water and drinking water, I use filtered water and have an under sink water filter...and also an activated charcoal filter takes out any residual compounds that are in the water." Tongzhang Zheng, D.Sc., Professor of Epidemiology at the Yale School of Medicine and Consultant to the World Health Organization says, "Purifying water is wonderful and I know many friends [who do this], including ourselves, and I am confident it is going be helpful to prevent you from exposures." University of Minnesota's Robert Turesky, Ph.D. says "Charcoal filters can effectively remove many of the organic chemicals in water." David Wheeler, Ph.D., Assistant Professor of Biostatistics at Virginia Commonwealth University's Massey Cancer Center says, "A good thing people can do is filter their water. Buy a good filter and filter all your tap water for drinking and cooking. Get the best filter that you can, the stage 3 filters are better than the stage 2 filters, which are very inexpensive, and will take out more things like pharmaceuticals in the water...Also, I have only heard good things about steam distillation for cleaning water...".

Indeed, many experts believe that steam distilled water is the purest, cleanest water. Ze'ev Ronai, Ph.D., Scientific Director of Sanford Burnham laboratory says, "Distilled water uses a relatively simple process that removes most of the contaminants." The basic principle is simply removing contaminants in water by boiling it and then condensing the water vapor back to pure water. The best systems use a two-step process in which contaminants that have a boiling point below that of water are vented off and those that have a boiling point above water stay behind as residue. George Yu, Ph.D., Associate Professor of Molecular and Cellular Biology at Clemson University says, "I think steam distillation is a good way to get pure water...which would help eliminate small molecule contaminants." Jay Thomas Sutliffe, Ph.D., Associate Professor of Public Health at Northern Arizona University says, "I personally think steam distilled water is the best and some critics will always jump up and say that you take out all the minerals and what I come back to is, 'I don't drink water to get my minerals, I eat fruits and vegetables and whole grains and legumes to get my minerals - I am not looking to my water supply to give me minerals...'". The World Health Organization concurs that the main source of minerals should be food, not water. A high quality multi-vitamin with minerals would be useful for anyone drinking steam distilled water if the individual has a concern about getting essential minerals. Northeastern State University's Dragos Albinescu, Ph.D. adds, "Steam distilled water is pure water." Melissa Davis, Ph.D., Assistant Professor of Genetics at the University of Georgia says, "I am definitely a fan of distilled water."

An example of an excellent company that utilizes a very high quality steam distillation process is Mountain Valley Spring Company based in Hot Springs National Park, Arkansas. They start with very clean spring water and purify it further through several steps including ozonation that destroys bacteria and other microorganisms and then steam distillation which removes other contaminants. They sell their distilled water to consumers under the trade name "Diamond" through distributors in sealed glass bottles that eliminates the possibility of the leaching of chemicals from plastic bottles. To find a distributor near you or to place on online order, visit the company's web site at www.mountainvalleyspring.com.

Eat Organic When Possible

A plan to keep environmental chemicals out of your body to the extent possible should include avoiding pesticides and other chemical additives in foods but most people are not doing that very well. Moffit Cancer Center's Thomas Sellers, Ph.D., M.P.H. says:

> I believe 100% that we should do everything we can to clear up the water supply, to avoid unhealthy additives to food, to improve the quality of the food supply because 'you are what you eat'. What I am concerned about is that we have the opportunity to take control and responsibility but Americans are not doing it.

Melinda Oberleitner, R.N., D.N.S, Associate Dean, College of Nursing and Allied Sciences at University of Louisiana adds, "An article in the Journal of Reproductive Toxicology points out that... more than 10,000 chemicals, are allowed to be added directly or indirectly to human food pursuant to the United States FDA amendment of 1958...Those are chemicals that preserve flavor, enhance taste or appearance, prevent spoilage, part of food packaging, and as of 2010, the FDA can't keep up with testing them anymore...". Northeastern State University's Dragos Albinescu, Ph.D. says, "I totally agree that avoiding herbicides and pesticides is a good thing from the point of view of human health... organic is much better...". University of Georgia's Melissa Davis, Ph.D. says, "Be vigilant about the products you consume and whenever possible, use organic - organic dairy products, organic produce - all of these things, we do know protect DNA at a molecular level...". Robert Amato, D.O., Chief of the Division of Oncology at Memorial Hermann Cancer Center says, "With an organic plant-based diet, there are less chemicals. Those chemicals can affect cells which can become foreign to your body and thus they are potentially cancer cells...".

At the same time, it's important to understand that not all organic foods are created equal. Alice Whittemore, Ph.D., Professor of Health Policy, Epidemiology and Biostatistics at Stanford University says, "A lot of things are called organic but whether they are really pesticide free is something else again." University of Pittsburgh's Thomas Kensler, Ph.D. points out that one cannot eliminate all risks and even people who eat organic food should consider that, "... the farm product that is growing under organic conditions doesn't mean that the field across the street doesn't use pesticides and some of it blows over or is in the groundwater." For those who choose organic, products grown in the US are generally preferable as they tend to follow more stringent standards in order to call something organic as opposed to other countries who standards and inspections may be more lax. USDA (United States Department of Agriculture) Certified Organic producers must follow rigorous standards to qualify for that designation and is recommended whenever such products are available. The USDA has strengthened its oversight of organic products, using methods such as inspections and residue testing to ensure the integrity of organic products from farm to market. In addition, USDA has also developed clear standards, investigates consumer complaints and takes action against farmers and businesses that violates the law. Anthony Shield, M.D., Associate Director of the Barbara Ann Karmanos Cancer Institute at Wayne State University says, "I think the US tends to be better...". Even within the United States, some states are better than others. California organic products, for example, have a good reputation for following strict organic guidelines. University of Iowa's Bill Fields, Ph.D., M.S. says, "California in many ways leads the way with trying to reduce exposures to pesticides and other toxins."

While we need more uniform standards in the US for food producers and retailers who advertise to consumers that products are organic, we should not let perfection get in the way of the good. Dartmouth Medical School's Angeline Andrew, Ph.D. notes, "Although it's difficult to know exactly what organic means...my personal opinion is that if the foods you buy are lower in pesticides and other harmful chemicals, then theoretically that would reduce exposure and be protective...". Northern Arizona University's Jay Thomas Sutliffe, Ph.D. adds, "I think it's a great idea...I just think that where there's more, what we call old-fashioned techniques used in farming such as rotating of crops and those types of things rather than the chemical farming...". It's probably a good idea whenever possible to purchase your organic food from reliable suppliers such as large grocery stores and high quality health food stores like Whole Foods. Wayne State University's Dr. Shield says, "I personally tend to choose organic...I would suggest organic...[but] you should be eating fruits and vegetables [whether organic or not]."

Eating organic is not only better for your health, but using natural farming processes is also better for the environment. Cleaning up our environment over the long run will reduce cancer risk throughout the US and the world. Joseph Ahlander, Ph.D., Assistant Professor of Biology at Northeastern State University says, "Regarding organic food, traces of pesticide may have a negative effect on human health but it's more of an environmental problem as far as I'm concerned." Henry Thompson, Ph.D., Professor of Agriculture at Colorado State University says about organic food, "...if you can afford it...it certainly is a fine choice and it's good for the environment to choose organic." Georgetown University's Laura Anderko, Ph.D., R.N. advises, "Go organic whenever you can afford it as there are fruits and vegetables that are likely to contain pesticides...". Wichita State University's William Hendry, Ph.D. notes, "There are some pesticides that are thought to be dangerous...so organic is not a bad idea." Wayne Sanderson, Ph.D., Professor and Chair of Epidemiology at the University of Kentucky adds, "... many of the pesticides that we are using have not been fully tested to determine their carcinogenic potentials." Melinda Irwin, Ph.D., Co-Director of the Cancer Prevention and Control Program at Yale University adds, "Fruits and vegetables are healthy and even healthier would be the organic fruits and vegetables." Virginia Commonwealth University's

David Wheeler, Ph.D. says that to reduce cancer risk, "...choose food that was not grown with pesticides. Choose organic produce and vegetables whenever possible."

It is also very important from a health standpoint to eat a wide variety of fruits and vegetables, whether you can afford organic or not, because of the protective qualities against cancer. If you cannot afford organic, just wash your fruits and vegetables and peel off the outer skin whenever possible. Abby Benninghoff, Ph.D., Assistant Professor of Epigenetics at Utah State University adds, "If there is concern about pesticides, wash and peel your fruits." Korry Hintze, Ph.D., Assistant Professor of Molecular Biology and Applied Agriculture and Nutrition at Utah State University says, "I have actually heard people say that they won't eat fruits and vegetables unless they are organic. The point I want to make is that I think the benefits of eating conventional fruits and vegetables for people who can't afford organic foods outweigh not eating any fruits and vegetables at all." Yawei Zhang, M.D., Ph.D., M.P.H., Associate Professor of Cancer Epidemiology at the Yale School of Medicine says, "There are often residual pesticides on the vegetables and fruit so wash them well and soak them in water...because many pesticides are water-soluble and it will help remove them...I generally let them soak for about an hour...".

Consumers also have to be on the lookout for meat and fish that have absorbed contaminants from their environments that are harmful to human health. Laura Anderko, Ph.D., R.N. echoes the advice of many nutrition experts saying, "Move away from meat... the less likely you will be to eat all kinds of contaminants whether antibiotics, steroids or pesticides." Thomas Sellers, Ph.D., M.P.H., Professor of Epidemiology at the Moffit Cancer Center says, "It's natural to think about the amount of...chemicals that get into the water supply which will then get into animals that we eat... so it's very reasonable to speculate that is a factor contributing to cancer". For example, while many types of fish can be part of a healthy diet as evidenced from the Japanese who have eaten a lot of fish and live relatively long lives, fish from polluted waters or eating too much of certain types of fish can cause harm. Christine Curran, Ph.D., Assistant Professor of Biology at Northern Kentucky University says:

> There are fatty fish that have high levels of PCBs...They are very hard to break down. They have been banned for decades but they persist in the environment - they resist degradation. You can still measure them in breast milk. Industrial areas like Ohio and Michigan sometimes post warnings that advise not to eat the fish because they have mercury and PCBs in them.

Bruce Ames, Ph.D., Professor Emeritus of Nutrition and Metabolism at the University of California, Berkeley adds, "I know two people, one a Nobel Prize winner, who ended up with mercury poisoning. They thought fish are good for you so they ate sword-fish every night and they both got mercury poisoning." Dr. David Wheeler adds, "People should avoid farm raised salmon because of increased levels of PCBs...which levels are 10 to 40 times higher than wild caught salmon. Instead, buy wild caught Alaskan salmon... and eat smaller fish that are down lower in the food chain that don't bio accumulate the PCBs as something like tuna or a larger fish would...People should probably not be eating fish every day, I don't think that would be wise."

Avoid BPAs and Phthalates

BPAs and phthalates were referenced earlier because there has been a lot of attention in the popular press and medical literature pertaining to the health risks of these environmental chemicals that are in plastic bottles, plastic bags, inside cans – in other words, all around us. An average household uses about 500 plastic bottles per year and the worldwide use is estimated at one trillion plastic bottles! Erin Eaton, Ph.D., Associate Professor of Biology at Francis Marion University explains:

> What people don't realize is our bodies are constantly being bombarded by carcinogens, chemicals that are inducing DNA damage...Just like with tobacco use and excessive alcohol use. Avoid chemicals, BPA's and these types of things...BPA's have been the big buzzword for the last five years or so.

University of Iowa's Bill Fields, Ph.D., M.S. points out that, "A lot of [these chemicals] are endocrine disruptors...a big area of research right now is endocrine disruptors and the hazards they pose...So many of these chemicals are synthetic and we don't know the long-term hazards...BPAs are suspected carcinogens...". Carlos Sonnenschein, M.D., Professor of Integrative Physiology and Pathobiology at Tufts University School of Medicine says we should try to avoid endocrine disrupters including those caused by "synthetic chemicals such as BPA that are pervasive in our environment." Often times, the plastics chemical industry will just replace one harmful chemical with another untested chemical that may be just as harmful. Anna Jeng, Ph.D., Associate Professor and Director of the School of Community and Environmental Health at Old Dominion University explains, "They use other synthetic compounds to replace BPAs that may be just as harmful, so that when they say, 'That's a BPA free bottle, it is safe to use' - don't believe that." Cecilia Williams, Ph.D., Assistant Professor of Biotechnology at the University of Houston says, "Try to avoid estrogen-like exposures...such as BPAs...Virtually everybody is exposed to BPA's and they have it in their blood."

The President's Cancer Panel also expressed concern about BPAs and phthalates stating:

> One such ubiquitous chemical, Bisphenol A [BPA] is still found in many consumer products and remains unregulated in the United States, despite the growing link between BPA and

several diseases, including various cancers. BPAs are found in many plastics including plastic bottles for soft drinks and plastic bags to hold food that are used by billions worldwide. Also, canned food or drink can contain BPAs which can leach into the drinks or food they contain before they are consumed. BPAs are known endocrine disrupters and studies have linked them to increased breast cancer risk and adult precancerous lesions in the pancreas. The endocrine disrupter nature of BPAs also appear to contribute to obesity which is a major risk factor for cancer. Studies conducted by the Centers for Disease Control found BPAs in the urine of 93% of children and adults tested. Phthalates have also been found in the urine of a high percentage of people studied and is a known risk factor for breast cancer. Phthalates are found in a variety of products including plastics bottles, vinyl, cosmetics, pharmaceuticals, medical devises, children's toys and detergents. Women may be at particularly high risk of phthalates due their links to breast cancer since phthalates are ubiquitous in cosmetic and personal care products.

Given the evidence regarding BPAs and phthalates, individuals should take steps to be sure they are avoiding products that contain these chemicals. As a starting point, consumers should stop drinking soft drinks out of plastic bottles and use glass or stainless steel containers to transport their favorite beverage. In addition, government needs to become more aggressive about regulating these chemicals. Northeastern State University's Joseph Ahlander, Ph.D. says, "There should be regulations to reduce BPAs given our understanding that it has a measurable impact on hormone function and metabolic function."

Virginia Commonwealth University's Dr. David Wheeler adds:

BPA's have been banned in the European Union and Canada for use in baby bottles. Now, in the US, I believe baby bottles and sippy cups are not made with BPA anymore but there is still a lot of BPA out there in plastic bottles in the US and metal cans are lined with BPA so it's not just the plastic bottles but if you are drinking a lot of canned soup then you are likely increasing your exposure to BPA.

Reduce Other Potentially Harmful Environmental Chemicals – In Your Own Home

It might surprise most people to discover that their homes are a repository for potentially harmful environmental chemicals in addition to those already mentioned that are common on food, in drinking water and in plastic bottles and bags. Those described below are among the more common toxins found in homes.

Flame Retardants

Many years ago, due to fires in homes, laws were created that mandated that flame retardant chemicals be added to lots of things that people have in their homes. University of South Carolina's John Vena, Ph.D., explains:

> Flame retardant chemicals, on the one hand reduce fires because they are used in carpets, furniture, etc...but at the same time they are ubiquitous in the environment and bio accumulate in us...These and many, many others that we use that can be beneficial on the one hand yet when they get into the environment are persistent and have adverse effects on us.

Some cancer experts avoid carpeting in their own homes because of the carcinogenic nature of the flame retardant chemicals. Yale School of Medicine's Yawei Zhang, M.D., Ph.D., M.P.H. says, "I don't have carpets in my house because of the toxic chemicals in flame retardants in carpeting." It's not just carpeting, CBS News found that 84% of couches in California homes contained harmful flame retardants and reported that, "It is troubling to see that a majority of homes have at least one flame retardant at levels beyond what the federal government says is safe."

Household Cleaning Chemicals

Almost all Americans have household cleaners in their homes that have potentially harmful chemicals. Toxicologists have a unique perspective on the issue of toxins including those in our homes and environment since they spend their entire professional lives studying such phenomena. Luoping Zhang, Ph.D., a toxicologist and Professor of Environmental Health Sciences at the University of California, Berkeley School of Public Health explains:

> You have to be aware what kind of exposures you have in your everyday life. For example, your household cleaning products...I tell my cleaning person not to use all the regular stuff, I will only allow her to use water and soap. Whenever you buy, you always have to read the labels and see what kind of chemicals they contain. For most people, they see the chemicals but still have no idea what toxins are carcinogenic that are in there. So, I would generally say, reduce any unnecessary man-made products.

Virginia Commonwealth University's David Wheeler adds, "Choose household products carefully...that are made with non-toxic substances...Use natural cleaning products in the house whenever possible...".

Formaldehyde

Formaldehyde, a known carcinogen, has been used for years in products such as pressed wood which many people have in their homes. A US Congressional investigation a few years ago found that formaldehyde was making people sick after the federal government put displaced residents in trailers due to Hurricane Katrina. The trailers were found to have pressed wood inside of them that contained formaldehyde in the glue that was causing the illness. Millions of Americans have similar products in their own homes including laminated or pressed wood that contains formaldehyde. Tim Byers, M.D., M.P.H., Associate Dean of Cancer Prevention and Control at the University of Colorado Cancer Center says about formaldehyde and proper ventilation in homes to reduce exposure:

> I really think we need to minimize the exposure [to formaldehyde]. We'll never get down to zero for that because it's used in the production of so many things but getting the dose down low is, I think, important...Risks are exacerbated because we are not circulating the air very well indoors...We have sealed our homes so well in order to not have much exchange of outside air with inside air...We try to improve our heat efficiency by sealing everything up...Economic pressures to save money on heating and air-conditioning by sealing our homes have had an adverse effect on indoor air quality.

Cosmetics and Underarm Deodorants

Cosmetics and underarm deodorants are among many personal care products that contain potentially harmful synthetic chemicals. Laura Anderko, Ph.D., R.N., Cancer Epidemiologist and Fellow at the Center for Social Justice at Georgetown University says, "With hygiene products, a lot of products that we utilize contain carcinogens such as shampoos, makeup, underarm deodorants...".

Laura Vanderberg, Ph.D., Professor of Environmental Health at University of Massachusetts School of Public Health Sciences adds:

...there are things in our personal care products like cosmetics...there are some very simple things that people can do to protect themselves from those types of chemicals...The more we use products that have chemicals, the more likely we are to be exposed to compounds that at really low doses increase our risk.

Virginia Commonwealth University's David Wheeler, Ph.D. adds, "Choose cosmetics that are naturally based and avoid cosmetics that have parabens in them...You can find these in a specialty grocery store that carry lots of organic products like Whole Foods...". For online shoppers, Amazon.com is a good source of USDA certified organic personal care products.

Miscellaneous Household Chemical Suggestions

Dr. Wheeler further suggests:

Avoid the use of plastics in food preparation and water storage. For example, use a stainless steel container or a glass container for storing water. Also, when storing food and heating up food in a microwave oven, use a glass or ceramic container...Choose household products carefully...that are made with non-toxic substances...Personally, I would avoid the use of non-stick pans for cooking as there is some concern that the chemicals in some pans used during cooking are being ultimately consumed by people...Reduce or eliminate pesticides and fertilizers used for landscaping. Many of these pesticides contain chemicals that are on the list of being suspected carcinogens...Avoid household products that have warnings on them, for example, a product has a known carcinogen in it. That sounds kind of obvious but I don't think most people look at that...There are a lot of products that contain possible, probable or known carcinogens that are used in everyday products...for example, 'The state of California has determined that a chemical used in this product is a known carcinogen'. In California, it has to be written as a warning on the bottle.

Reduce Chemical Exposures in Your Workplace

In addition to our own homes, there are cancer risks from environmental chemical substances at places of employment for millions of Americans. For example, in the healthcare industry, which employs well over 11 million Americans, radiation and hazardous chemicals are used that potentially increase risk exposure. The World Health Organization (WHO) points to cancer risks from industrial processes as well such as aluminum and coke production, iron and steel founding and rubber manufacturing. They further estimate that about 125 million people in the world are exposed to asbestos in the workplace and more than 107,000 people die each year from asbestos related lung cancer, mesothelioma and asbestosis resulting from occupational exposures. University of Kansas Medical Center's John Neuberger, Dr. P.H. cautions, "If you are doing any remediation around your house, be careful of any exposures to asbestos if there is any in the house. When you knock it about it might get in the air and then you would be inhaling it and sometimes that happens in the workplace as well." The World Health Organization estimates that one in three deaths from occupational cancer is caused by asbestos.

In the United States, the Occupational Safety and Health Administration (OSHA) is tasked with assuring the safest workplace possible for American workers and they may not be keeping up as they should given all of the new research on environmental chemical exposures that occur not just in peoples' homes, but in the workplace. Karl Kelsey, M.D., M.P.H., Professor of Community Health and Director of the Center for Environmental Health at Brown University notes, "It has been a long time since, for example, the Occupational Safety and Health Administration promulgated any new regulatory framework for the protection of workers."

Additional protection for farmers, for example, may well be in order as they often work with large amounts of pesticides putting them at higher risk of developing cancer. For example, Plymouth State University's Barbara McCahan, Ph.D. says that pesticides used on pineapples in Hawaii found their way into the water table and water supplies of the farmers there affecting them and their families adding, "...farm workers that were using the pesticides - it was really significantly impacting their fertility and even the wives of those farmworkers who were not actually in the fields but were drinking the water in those areas - their fertility levels were being impacted." Other studies show similar results. Linda Birnbaum, Ph.D., Director of the National Institute of Environmental Health Science says of a large study involving farmers who use pesticides, "...we are seeing an association between quite a number of different pesticides and certain types of cancer as well as other health effects."

If in your workplace, you suspect that you are coming into contact with hazardous materials or other risks that can be remediated, do some research on your own and call the Occupational Health and Safety Administration for advice on how best to protect yourself and your coworkers.

Precautionary Principle, Public Policy and Reducing Risk of Environmental Chemicals: Follow the Lead of the European Union and Overhaul the Toxic Substances Control Act

Up until now, the Precautionary Principle has been discussed in terms of the approach that individuals and families should take to protect their health and minimize cancer risk by reducing exposure to synthetic environmental chemicals. However, University of Massachusetts' Laura Vanderberg, Ph.D. says the Precautionary Principle not only makes sense for individuals and families, but should be expanded saying:

I think the Precautionary Principle should also be applied at a societal level. If there is some evidence to suggest that chemicals used in a personal-care product can interfere with hormone signaling, why are they there? Why are we allowing companies to put these chemicals into things that we rub on our babies bodies? The Precautionary Principle applied at that level would say that we have to change the burden of proof and the burden of safety back to the people who are making these chemicals. I like the Precautionary Principle. I like the idea that once we know enough, we know enough. We don't have to prove something and we don't need to get to the same level we did with tobacco that took decades to prove that something was dangerous.

The President Cancer Panel Report states that:

Weak laws and regulations, inefficient enforcement, regulatory complexity, and fragmented authority allow avoidable exposures to known or suspected cancer-causing and cancer-promoting agents to continue to proliferate in the workplace and the community...Enforcement of most existing regulations is poor...Industry has exploited regulatory weakness such as government's reactionary approach to regulation...A precautionary, prevention oriented approach should replace current reactionary approaches to environmental contaminants in which human harm must be proven before action is taken to reduce or eliminate exposure.

Keith Wailoo, Ph.D., Professor at the Woodrow Wilson School of Public Affairs at Princeton University adds, "In the last 30 years we have had a very industry friendly approach to regulation that has, in some ways, tied the hands of regulators...with regards to all of these sorts of substances...We just don't have the resources, we had a policy of kind of starving regulations, starving government to prevent it from actually doing its job of protecting the public health in these kinds of cases." University of South Carolina's John Vena, Ph.D. adds:

> When there are potential adverse effects, then it only makes sense to be precautionary, address it and try to prevent the exposure to it, to use common sense until we know differently...The President's Cancer Panel Report was a warning to us that we need to be cognizant that most cancers are related to the environment and we need to be vigilant to address them.

The federal law that is supposed to protect the public from potentially harmful environmental chemicals is the Toxic Substances Control Act. It was passed more than 35 years ago and a number of public health organizations want to see it amended or replaced because it does not require testing of the vast majority of synthetic chemicals that are permitted to be marketed to millions of Americans. Among those wanting changes in the law are the American Academy of Pediatrics, the American Public Health Association, Physicians for Social Responsibility, American Medical Association, American Nurses Association, US Public Interest Research Group, Environmental Defense Fund, Lung Cancer Alliance and Asbestos Disease Awareness Association. Many individual health experts also believe the outdated law needs an overhaul. Brown University's Karl Kelsey, M.D. says:

> The Toxic Substances Control Act was promulgated in 1976...The problem is a big one as we have trouble testing as many chemicals as are made. The Congress in our public policy has been remiss in not reevaluating the situation...in its obligation to protect people I think has really been somewhat lax in recent years.

Georgetown University's Laura Anderko, Ph.D., R.N. adds, "We need a stronger chemicals policy and the President's Cancer Panel made pretty strong statements about that. The Toxic Substances Control Act is outdated and not doing the job that Americans think it's doing. Is the government protecting us? Not really"

Many believe that the US should have a chemical testing program more similar to the European Union which has a totally different, and better, approach from a public health policy perspective.

Christine Curran, Ph.D., Assistant Professor of Biology at Northern Kentucky University says of Europe's chemical testing legislation, "Europe and the REACH program looks at these a little differently...Its Registration, Evaluation, Authorization of Chemicals.. It is generally considered more conservative in some ways." Virginia Commonwealth University's David Wheeler, Ph.D. explains:

> In the United States, the regulation process is a reactionary one which is counter to the Precautionary Principle regulation system in the European Union. In order for a product to be banned in the United States, there needs to be a huge amount of evidence that shows without any doubt that a chemical will cause cancer in humans. There is a long list of chemicals that are suspected to be cancer-causing to humans that are used on a daily basis in the US. It takes a long time in the US for a product to be found to be so horrible that it is banned like DDT and PCBs which were banned in the 1970s or 80s in the United States...The key difference between the United States and European Union system is that the burden of proof for showing that a chemical is harmful to humans, falls on the producer of the chemical in the EU where in the United States, basically most of the chemicals are released into the products and general population without a lot of testing and it's only after years of studies being done, studies on risk in the population, that shows that there's a significant amount of increased risk using that substance that it might be banned...

University of Pittsburgh's Thomas Kensler, Ph.D. says the European Union "requires more information up front before they make a decision to allow a material into the marketplace...forward-looking and predictive science is a reasonable approach." Utah State University's Abby Benninghoff, Ph.D. points out that:

> Europe uses the Precautionary Principle where you must prove a compound is safe before you can sell it on the market. In the United States, it is the opposite, you must prove harm before you can restrict a compound's use...The problem in the US is that it is a very high burden of proof, to prove harm and to prove specific harm...Speaking as an American who was exposed like my fellow citizens...we can certainly do better to protect people from this kind of potential harm.

Dr. Wheeler adds, "I think that the European Union model generally protects the population better than the US model. In the past, there were many chemicals that were assumed to be safe, for example, DDT or PCBs and these substances have now been banned after decades of use...We are unnecessarily increasing cancer risk for millions of people by not using the Precautionary Principle system...". Carlos Crespo, Ph.D., Professor of Community Health at Portland State University explains:

> In Europe, a chemical is considered guilty until proven innocent. In the US, chemicals are innocent until proven guilty... It's not until you show that, 'Oh yeah that stuff is starting to kill people' and by the time you can fix that, you have built an industry that is going to protect that chemical from being regulated instead of the other way around, having to prove that a chemical is not going to cause harm in the population before you actually mass use it. Look how hard it is to get BPA out of baby bottles. It has been done piecemeal from one state to another and it's so difficult to convince

legislators that it is the right thing to do...We cannot trust industry to police itself. They have a conflict of interest.

Testing Synthetic Chemicals

In a way, when it comes to synthetic chemicals, scientists and health advocates have been fighting with one hand tied behind their backs with the deck definitely stacked against them. It takes a long time to prove that a chemical causes harm to human health, combined with weak regulations in the US and a chemical industry that is adding thousands of new chemicals to the marketplace in rapid-fire succession. It is a recipe for disaster and individual Americans and their families are paying the price with increased cancer risk and, in too many cases, the development of cancers within those families.

In addition to overhauling the Toxic Substances Control Act, improved methodologies for testing synthetic chemicals has the potential to more rapidly identify carcinogenic substances in the future. The National Institute of Environmental Health's Linda Birnbaum, Ph.D. explains:

> We now have 240 chemicals that are listed as known human carcinogens or reasonably anticipated to be human carcinogens...We are in fact leading part of the effort called Tox 21 - which is really Toxicology in the 21st Century...and what we are doing is trying to turn toxicology into a predictive mode, a predictive science and part of what we are doing is developing rapid and high and medium throughput methods to test high volumes of chemicals in a relatively short period of time. So far, what this is doing for us is allowing us to identify chemicals for which we have a much higher concern... about 10% [of all chemicals]...and put them into the more traditional testing processes that helps to prioritize what is it that we really want to test...Many of these chemicals are

known as endocrine disruptors...which have the potential to cause cancer.

There are certainly some limitations to current chemical testing methodologies. While chemicals are usually tested one at a time, advances may also need to be made to determine how chemicals will interact with others in the human body since in the real world, they are not in our bodies in isolation. Dr. Kensler says that some chemicals may:

> ...pose modest risks by themselves but in concert with others they could become important so an area where we need more information and better understanding is the notion of complex mixtures and reactions between chemicals. Our programs are completely designed to test chemicals one by one by one but in the real world they don't work one by one by one. That's an area where we may look backwards and say, 'We missed some important concepts and exposures.'

Edward Trapido, Ph.D., Professor and Chair of Epidemiology at the Louisiana School of Public Health adds, "We tend to test compounds in isolation rather than in combination and in fact that is not how you are exposed to them...For example, people who smoke and drink alcohol are at a very elevated risk of oral cancer and upper respiratory cancers."

7

Other Risk Factors for Cancer

Radon

Unlike most of the other environmental chemicals found in your home described above, radon is naturally occurring, found in many American homes and very dangerous. Residential exposure to radon gas from soil and building materials is the second leading cause of lung cancer after tobacco smoke. University of Iowa's Bill Fields, Ph.D., M.S. points out that, "People don't realize that radon is the leading environmental cause of cancer mortality in the United States." Wallace Akerley, M.D., a medical oncologist and Director of Thoracic Oncology at the Huntsman Cancer Institute at the University of Utah who is one of the foremost experts on the health effects of radon in the US explains:

> Radon is a naturally occurring gas which causes lung cancer...there's this huge lack of awareness...half of the country has relatively high radon levels. In my state, one out of three tests come up with an elevated level of radon that the EPA says you should fix...Your house is supposed to be a safe haven not a place to get a cancer. Radon is a naturally occurring, colorless, odorless radioactive gas - it is uranium essentially in the earth...The EPA has mapped it out and pretty much the northern half of the United States has elevated radon levels with some states higher than others. So, there is radioactive material in the earth, it's a gas and it percolates

up...In our new world we have the super insulated houses that hold in whatever is there to keep our heat present... Radon leaks out of the ground and mixes into the air...in your house and you can't see it, smell it or otherwise know it but if you measure it, it is relatively easy to fix and relatively inexpensive. Radon is probably responsible for 18,000 to 20,000 deaths in the US per year making it the seventh leading cause of all cancer deaths in America...I take care of patients in the clinic with lung cancer and more than half the patients I see say, 'I don't drink, I don't smoke and yet I have lung cancer, what's all this about?'. We believe radon is responsible for a large fraction of the lung cancers here among non-smokers. Research shows it is the number one cause of non-smokers lung cancer. You can test for radon in your house and it only cost about $30-$40 to run the test. You put a canister in your basement or lowest level of your house if there is no basement and you leave it there for 48 hours and then you send it in to a certified laboratory that will analyze it and tell you whether your radon level is excessive or not. The fix is easy. If you measure it and it's not there, you feel good. If you measure it and it is there, there are relatively inexpensive ways to patch it or to run a pipe and vent it away from your living quarters.

Virginia Commonwealth University's David Wheeler, Ph.D. concurs adding, "Radon is a big factor for lung cancer so as a homeowner, I would manage radon levels within the home. If a person is thinking about buying a home, you should have the radon levels checked in that house." University of Kansas Medical Center's John Neuberger, Dr. P.H. says, "Your contractor can test the radon level in your home and if it is above the EPA guidelines, mediate your home because radon does have the capacity to damage your lungs as it decays." It would also be wise for any homeowner or potential homeowner to do some research about the risk of radon in his or her community and state. Some states are proactive in working with its citizens. Keith Wailoo, Ph.D., Professor at the Woodrow Wilson School of Public Affairs at Princeton University says, "In New Jersey, there is a radon abatement system in place. In areas where radon is naturally occurring, when you purchase a new house, you will often have an assessment done...".

Air Pollution

Another very significant health hazard and cancer risk in the US and throughout the world is air pollution. The air that we breathe, for all too many people, has become another significant source of synthetic chemical substances that enter our bodies. As noted earlier, air pollution has recently been declared to be a known carcinogen by the International Agency for Research on Cancer. The air quality index in many cities in America receives poor marks putting their residents at cancer risk. Peter Shields, M.D., a medical oncologist and Deputy Director of the James Cancer Center at Ohio State University says, "The International Agency for Research on Cancer just classified air pollution as a cause of lung cancer following many, many different studies...I think they did a great job. They looked at a lot of high-quality studies." Joshua Muscat, Ph.D., an Epidemiologist and Professor of Health Science at the Penn State Cancer Institute concurs saying, "There is a growing body of evidence that seems to be indicating that air pollution is associated with increased rates of cancer...". University of Texas Medical School's Robert Amato, D.O. adds:

> The air we breathe...if you live in Houston, where I'm from, we have the oil and gas industry and you go down that corridor and you see the pollutants in the air and then you realize patients are coming from that area with predominant lung cancer, bladder cancer. Why? Is it them or is it the air they are exposed to? It's the environment.

Virginia Commonwealth University's David Wheeler, Ph.D. explains:

> With air pollution, of course, there will be variation in the exposure level that is thought to have a dose response relationship between air pollution and certain cancer risks. Obviously, the more air pollution you have the greater burden your body will face for cancer risk. People should try to limit their exposure to air pollution, if possible. There is certainly a great deal of variation of air pollution in the US which not only varies by location, but varies by time within any given location. For example, there are increases in air pollution during rush hour so if someone could avoid being outside and breathing the polluted air during rush hour, that would be a positive thing.

Xiaohui Xu, M.D., Ph.D., M.P.H., Professor of Environmental Epidemiology at the University of Florida explains that public policies can reduce air pollution but explains that:

> People who live in cities are going to be exposed to more air pollution...Air pollution is everywhere but to varying degrees with some areas having high levels of pollution and some relatively low...The EPA has a very reliable daily air quality reporting system so if you know that today is going to be a highly polluted air day, you could avoid outdoor exercise during rush hour which can help reduce your exposure to the air pollution...pay attention to the EPA data on fine particulate matter which can penetrate deep in your lungs and hazardous substances from air pollution that can get into your blood...and use air filters in your home...

In the modern world, much of our air pollution is manmade coming from our automobiles and other modes of transportation that use fossil fuels, industrial production and coal burning for electrical generation. This is truly a global problem. It has been estimated that Los Angeles in the coming years will have trouble meeting established air-quality standards due to development in China. Why? The United States and China are the two largest emitters of greenhouse gases and the air pollution from those two countries and many others circulates through the atmosphere around the globe. University of Utah's Wallace Akerley, M.D. says of air pollution problems in America and throughout the developed world, "Bad air, cars, carbon monoxide and other chemicals are being put out by industry and I do think as time goes by, we will have to make some serious judgments. Do we want personal freedoms of driving and weigh that against the risks and potential benefits of moving toward public transportation." Tufts University School of Medicine's Carlos Sonnenschein, M.D. says that the pollution that we are creating today to make our lives easier is degrading the environment, increasing our cancer risk and points out that, "Our grandchildren are going to pay for many of the things that we are enjoying today so if we take the long view, we have to be careful about what we enjoy today so we don't jeopardize future generations."

For now, however, some strategies you can implement to protect yourself and your family from air pollution include limiting outdoor activity on bad air quality days, living in a rural area or city with a good air quality index and purchasing the best air filters for your home that you can afford. People spend a lot of time in their own homes – about one-third of their time sleeping plus additional time for non-sleeping and weekend relaxation time so a home filtration strategy is important to reduce exposures. This relates directly to the earlier point pertaining to reducing our dose of any environmental toxin as part of a wellness and anti-cancer strategy. In addition, the American Lung Association suggests the following tips to reduce exposure to air pollution for you and your family:

1. Check daily air-quality levels and air pollution forecasts in your area. Sources include local radio and TV weather reports, newspapers and online at www.epa.gov/airnow.

2. Use less energy in your home. Generating electricity and other sources of energy creates air pollution. By reducing energy use, you can help improve air quality, curb greenhouse gas emissions and save money.

3. Avoid exercising outdoors when pollution levels are high. When the air is bad, walk indoors in a shopping mall or gym or use an exercise machine. Always avoid exercising near high-traffic areas. Limit the amount of time your child spends playing outdoors if the air quality is unhealthy.

4. Encourage your child's school to reduce school bus emissions. Most buses use heavily polluting diesel engines. Newer fuels and engines are cleaner. To keep exhaust levels down, schools should not allow school buses to idle outside of their buildings.

5. Walk, bike or carpool. Combine trips. Use buses, subways, light rail systems, commuter trains or other alternatives to driving your car.

6. Fill up your gas tank after dark. Gasoline emissions evaporate as you fill up your gas tank. These emissions contribute to the formation of ozone, a component of smog. Fill up after dark to keep the sun from turning those gases into air pollution.

7. Don't burn wood or trash. Burning firewood and trash are among the major sources of particulate pollution (soot) in many parts of the country. If you must use a fireplace or stove for heat, convert woodstoves to natural gas, which produces far fewer emissions.

8. Use hand powered or electric lawn care equipment rather than gasoline powered. Two-stroke engines like lawnmowers and leaf or snow blowers often have no pollution control devices. They can pollute the air even more than cars.

9. Don't allow anyone to smoke indoors and support measures to make all public places smoke-free. Dangerous particles from cigarette smoke can remain in the air long after the cigarette has been extinguished.

10. Get involved. Review your community's air pollution plans that support state and local efforts to clean up the air. Contact your local American lung Association at www.lung.org or at 1-800-586-4872 (1-800-LUNG-USA).

Get Adequate Sleep to Strengthen Your Immune System to help Fight off Cancer

Adequate sleep plays a very important role in achieving and maintaining good health and preventing cancer by strengthening the immune system. Experts say that we need seven or eight hours of sleep every night. Penn State's Joshua Muscat, Ph.D. says we can reduce our risk of developing cancer and other chronic diseases "by trying to get eight hours of sleep a night." Strengthening the immune system with adequate sleep and a healthy lifestyle is an important reason why many people can stay relatively healthy throughout much of their lives and stay strong enough to fight off many diseases that they might have contracted otherwise.

Certainly, our immune system often does a great job fighting off many potential illnesses. Lynette Phillips, Ph.D., Assistant Professor of Epidemiology at Kent State University says, "I think our bodies are tougher than we think." But to maintain that "toughness" we have to do our part. Most people have experienced times when they were weak and run-down from overwork, stress, unhealthy living and a lack of sleep which contributed to colds, flus and other illnesses. Anything that compromises our immune system also puts us at increased risk for illnesses, including cancer. Dale Shepard, M.D., Ph.D., a medical oncologist with the Cleveland Clinic says, "There's a number of things coming out that suggests that not sleeping enough can be linked to a lot of different things and cancer is certainly in that category...". University of North Florida's Cindy Battie, Ph.D. says, "The health of the immune system plays a big role which was shown in the HIV epidemic...showed us how important it is to have a strong immune system to fight cancer." Clemson University's Charlie Wei, Ph.D. says, "A healthy lifestyle will enhance your immune system activity even for people who have been diagnosed with cancer...". A healthy immune system can handle many gene mutations that otherwise could initiate cancer. Erin Eaton, Ph.D., Associate Professor of Biology at Francis Marion University explains, "Mutations occur daily but most mutations are taken care of by our immune system."

This is not to suggest that sleep alone is sufficient to maintain a strong immune system but it must be in conjunction with other healthy living strategies such as a healthy diet, managing stress and plenty of exercise – such a combination is the best way to maintain a healthy immune system. Conversely, insufficient sleep and sleep disorders contribute to a range of problems including poor work performance, driving accidents, relationship problems, anger management issues and health risks with links to a number of diseases, including cancer. Cheryl Jursyk, Ph.D., Professor of Biology at Boise State University says, "The better your immune system, the better you can fight things off." Old Dominion University's Richard Heller, Ph.D. adds, "It is our immune system that often protects us against cancer...the healthier you are...both physically and mentally, the better your immune system is." Often, sleep deficits are related to how we live including too much caffeine, nicotine, alcohol and stress from work or working on the home computer until the second we go to sleep. If you become aware that you snore and gasp for breath at night while trying to sleep, you should talk to your physician about being checked for sleep apnea, a serious but treatable medical condition. Sleep apnea affects 15 million American adults and is a chronic condition in which people who have it are unaware that they stop breathing for very short periods of time, up to hundreds of times per night.

If you are not getting sufficient sleep, try these tips from the National Sleep Foundation:

<u>10 Tips on How to Get Good Sleep</u>

1. Maintain a regular bed and wake time schedule including weekends.

2. Establish regular, relaxing bedtime routines such as soaking in a hot bath and then reading a book or listening to soothing music.

3. Create a sleep environment that is dark, quiet, comfortable and cool.

4. Sleep on a comfortable mattress and pillows.

5. Use your bedroom only for sleep and sex.

6. Finish eating at least 2 to 3 hours before your regular bedtime.

7. Exercise regularly. It is best to complete your workout at least a few hours before bedtime.

8. Avoid caffeine from coffee, tea, soft drinks and chocolate close to bedtime as they can keep you awake.

9. Avoid nicotine (i.e., cigarettes, tobacco products) since using these close to bedtime can lead to poor sleep.

Reduce Stress to the Extent Possible and Care for Your Mental Health

Stress is a normal part of life and everybody has it to one degree or another. It has likely always been part of the human condition. Humans evolved with stress. Undoubtedly, hunter-gatherers had to worry about finding food to survive. Later, subsistence farmers had to worry about sufficient crops to feed themselves and their families. While most people in the developed world have enough food for the day, pressures that cause stress are still present but just of a different nature. Lorraine Reitzel, Ph.D., Professor of Psychology at the University of Iowa says, "Everybody's lives right now are so busy and so stressful...".

Many health experts believe that excessive levels of stress can contribute to physical health problems, including cancer. For example, University of Missouri School of Medicine's Paul Dale, M.D. says:

> Stress seems to play an important role in cancer development. I have seen patients go 20 years cancer free and then have a major stressor in their life - their spouse dies, or their house burns down or they get fired and the original melanoma is back. It could have something to do with our immune system or immune surveillance and perhaps cancer formation or cancer recurrence...I tell patients, reduce stress if you can. It allows your body to work a lot better.

Barbara McCahan, Ph.D., Professor of Health and Physical Education at Plymouth State University Center for Active Living adds, "Probably the perception of stress in people's lives and what that does to them hormonally is also a big contributor to being overweight or obese."

The issue may be how much stress one has and how well it is managed that matters the most. Penn State's Joshua Muscat, Ph.D. says:

Stress has a big impact on the immune system. One person's stress level may be different than another person's stress level. There are competing theories. Some people think that a little bit of stress, is actually adaptive. Other people think that stress is harmful. It might be a matter of degree. A certain amount of stress might be actually protective but too much stress may be harmful to us and that may vary from individual to individual. One person's high stress threshold may be different than another person's.

University of Texas Medical School's Robert Amato, D.O. explains:

Reducing stress in your life, we all have it...we don't live in a stress free society...we wake up with stress, 'It's foggy outside' and that's immediate stress because now I have to drive to work in the dense fog. That's stress but how you deal with it - you exercise, get plenty of sleep and take care of your body so that you are reducing that stress burden.

Cancer experts say that reducing stress and improving mental health can help reduce your risks of cancer. Yale's Yawei Zhang, M.D., Ph.D. M.P.H. says:

I always tell my friends, be happier...That is very important. We know that lifestyle and environment is related to human cancer and I think psychosocial factors also play a major role. If you are a very positive person, you are always happy, it relieves some stress. If you have something stressful going on in your life, talk to your friends. Excessive stress can impact your immune system.

Oklahoma State University's Rashmi Kaul, Ph.D. adds, "Being happy and reducing stress is an important anticancer ingredient."

The American Mental Health Association and other experts offer the following mental health tips:

1. First and foremost, if you are suffering from depression, anxiety or any other mental health issue, seek the help of a professional such as a psychologist or other counselor and be sure to tell your primary care physician. Under the Affordable Care Act, mental health coverage is one of the 10 essential health benefits - use it if needed.

2. Value yourself. Treat yourself with kindness and respect, and avoid self-criticism. Everyone has traits they do not like about themselves. Do not let others define you - you are a beautiful and unique person. Take stock of the qualities you like about yourself, your accomplishments, your abilities and things you have to be grateful for in your life - make a written list of these and keep them in a handy place and look at them periodically when you are feeling down.

3. Relax. Take some time every day to relax, reflect and rejuvenate. Try meditating, taking a walk in a natural setting, reaching out spiritually or through prayer if you are religious person.

4. Make a plan. Decide what tasks you need to complete for the week and make a plan for when and how to do them. If you are overscheduled, decide what can wait a week or two. If you do not have much on your schedule, plan some activities that you will look forward to and help someone in need - you will feel good about it.

5. Surround yourself with supportive people. Make plans with family members and friends, or seek out activities in which you can meet new people, such as a club, class or support

group. Reconnect with someone you have lost touch with and create new memories.

6. Take care of your body. Taking care of yourself physically can improve your mental health as well.

7. If you have children, give them unconditional love, frequent praise and avoid sarcasm. Children need to know that your love does not depend on their accomplishments. Avoid physical punishment - explain the correct behaviors to your children and set the example. Praise and encourage them to help their self-esteem. Set realistic goals for them. Great parents put their children's needs before their own.

8. Be honest about your own mistakes – that's how we learn to do better the next time and to become better people.

9. Instead of turning to destructive behaviors in dealing with stress such as alcohol, over-eating or smoking, try vigorous exercise and confronting problems head-on and doing everything possible to solve the problems in your life that are causing the stress. For example, if you are under financial stress, do the best you can to cut unnecessary expenses or try to find ways to increase your income.

Get Vaccinated Against Certain Cancers

While there are not vaccines to protect against most cancers, as mentioned earlier, there are vaccines to protect against some liver cancers and cervical cancer. Several viruses are linked with these cancers which has led to the development of the vaccines. University of Pittsburgh's Thomas Kensler, Ph.D. says, "Cervical cancers and liver cancers are eminently preventable ones with the universal vaccination program against Hepatitis B virus and liver cancer." However, experts point out that the vaccines can only help prevent infections if they are given before the person is exposed to the cancer promoting virus.

A few types of the Human Papilloma Viruses (HPVs) are the main cause of cervical cancer in women, which is the second most common cancer among women worldwide. Although cervical cancer has become much rarer in the United States thanks to PAP tests which can detect precancerous changes in the cells of the cervix which can then be treated or removed. University of South Carolina's John Vena, Ph.D., says, "Every single boy and girl should be getting the HPV vaccine to prevent cancer later on not only for cervical cancer but other cancers that have been traced to the Human Papilloma Virus." Anthony Alberg, Ph.D., M.P.H., Professor of Public Health at the Medical University of South Carolina adds, "A major breakthrough in cancer prevention has been in the identification of the Human Papilloma Virus which causes cervical and other cancers. There is now an efficacious vaccine available for that. If you have teenagers, get them vaccinated, both boys and girls."

There are also vaccines to treat Hepatitis-B virus but not for Hepatitis-C, although other new drugs are available that can help significantly with the latter. Hepatitis-B virus and Hepatitis-C virus are linked to one third of liver cancers in the United States. The number is much higher in some other countries. Of the two viruses, Hepatitis-B is more likely to cause symptoms such as flulike symptoms or jaundice than Hepatitis-C that arises in people who do not even know they have the disease. University of Arizona's Peter Lance, M.D. says, "If we look around the world, actually one of the really common cancers is in fact liver cancer due to Hepatitis B virus. Now, part of regular vaccinations is everybody should be getting vaccinated against Hepatitis B virus." In the United States, the Hepatitis-B vaccine is recommended for all children and for adults who are at risk of exposure including people who have sex with more than one partner, injection drug users, prisoners, people in certain group homes, people with certain medical conditions, and certain high risk occupations for exposures such as healthcare workers.

If You Drink Alcohol, Do So in Moderation

The World Health Organization (WHO) says alcohol use is a risk factor for many cancer types including cancer of the oral cavity, pharynx, larynx, esophagus, liver, colorectal and breast. The Centers for Disease Control says that a large number of studies provide strong evidence that drinking alcohol is a risk factor for liver cancer. More than 100 studies have found an increased risk of breast cancer with increasing alcohol intake; and, colorectal cancer has been reported in more than 50 studies. They note that the risk of cancer increases with the amount of alcohol consumed.

The federal guidelines for those who drink alcohol are no more than one drink per day for women and two drinks per day for men. According to the National Cancer Institute, "Having more than two drinks each day for many years increases the risk of liver cancer and certain other cancers." Dean Hosgood, Ph.D., M.P.H., at Albert Einstein College of Medicine says, "When it comes to alcohol consumption, do it in moderation." Marc Schenker, M.D., M.P.H., Professor and Chair, Department of Public Health Science and Medicine at the University of California, Davis explains:

> [The cancer risk] is only in larger amounts. Not only that, but small amounts might be beneficial to your health. One drink a day may reduce the risk of certain chronic diseases except in the situation where you have a problem with alcohol. It is different than, let's say, cigarettes or asbestos in which even small amounts can be hazardous.

Louisiana State University's Edward Trapido, Ph.D. concurs saying, "Alcohol is related to several cancers such as liver cancer and breast cancer. Limit alcohol to a moderate amount...consumption in moderation has some benefit…". However, there is some research that shows that even small amounts of alcohol can increase cancer risk. Portland State University's Carlos Crespo, Ph.D. says that even though there is some evidence that says moderate amounts of alcohol may help from a cardiovascular standpoint, "For cancer, it's zero alcohol, the lower the risk. A little bit of alcohol, you increase your risk. It seems that there is a linear relationship…". Jay Thomas Sutliffe, Ph.D., Associate Professor of Public Health at Northern Arizona University says, "Alcohol in all your nutrition books is classified as a toxin…For me…I don't think I want to take in toxins."

The World Health Organization says that every year, alcohol kills 2.5 million people, including 320,000 young people between 15 and 29 years of age. They note it is the third leading risk factor for poor health globally, and excessive use of alcohol is responsible for almost 4% of all deaths in the world. The risk from heavy drinking for several cancer types substantially increases for people who are also heavy smokers. As we all know, some people drink so heavily and frequently that they become alcoholics. According to the University of Maryland Medical Center web site, "Genetic factors are significant in alcoholism and may account for about half of the total risk for alcoholism…However, genes alone do not determine whether someone will become alcohol dependent. Environment, personality and psychological factors also play a strong role." Alcohol dependence causes physiological changes in the heavy user of alcohol. Erin Eaton, Ph.D., Associate Professor of Biology at Francis Marion University explains, "With long-term use of alcohol, we have a change in our neurochemistry that causes delirium tremens, DTs, the nervous system becomes overexcited and that craving for alcohol to get the body back to what it has established as a baseline."

Mark Doescher, M.D., Professor of Family Medicine and Program Leader in Cancer Health Disparities at the University of Oklahoma Health Sciences Center says physicians like himself need to identify and address drinking problems with patients due to the associated health risks explaining:

> We have to give strong attention to alcohol for a variety of reasons and cancer is one of those - cancer of the esophagus, G.I. tract, etc...and for people who really have alcohol dependence, liver disease and cirrhosis...Having moderate amounts of wine or spirits is probably okay and may even be somewhat beneficial from a cardiac perspective but for a lot of patients they are unable to stop at a moderate amount of alcohol...A question I might ask is, 'Are you feeling guilty about it or do you think it's too much?' as it allows them to reflect about where they're at in their life and whether they think they have a problem so it opens up the door to be able to talk about it more freely as an issue?

Psychologists can also provide insight and assistance to people with drinking problems as well as to their families. David LaPorte, Ph.D., Professor of Psychology at Indiana University of Pennsylvania comments on the physiological aspects of alcoholism and how family members might help,

> People who are alcoholics get a different kind of buzz out of it than the rest of us who are able to stop at one, or at most two beers. We are fine with that and they are not. There is clearly something biological going on in their brain that is not going on in the rest of us...For that particular brain it may be that there is a much stronger basic biological or neural drive to consume that alcohol which of course is going to make it very difficult to get them to stop. There is this vicious cycle when people drink with their serotonin levels in that they get the immediate buzz from it which makes them feel good. The trouble is if you chronically abuse alcohol, it will deplete your serotonin storage which is why depression is one of the most common long-term outcomes of alcohol

abuse...The advice to family members who want to help [whether the problem is drinking, overeating or smoking] is to talk to the individual and say, 'I see what you're doing. What do you want me to do? What would be helpful to you?' Then, do what the person says is most helpful to him or her.

So, when it comes to alcohol, if you don't drink, think twice before starting as the risks of alcohol may well outweigh the benefits. If you already drink, stay within the federal guidelines of no more than one drink per day for women and two drinks per day for men. If you are regularly drinking beyond that, talk to your primary care physician or a professional counselor.

Preventing Skin Cancer

According to the Centers for Disease Control, skin cancer is the most common form of cancer in the United States which comes from too much exposure to ultraviolet rays from the sun and tanning salons. Bill Fields, Ph.D., M.S., Professor of Epidemiology at the University of Iowa says, "The primary cause of environmental cancer is sunlight...not mortality, but cancers overall...". Erin Eaton, Ph.D., Associate Professor of Biology at Francis Marion University explains:

> The evidence is incontrovertible...avoid prolonged exposure...for example, white people in Australia have extraordinarily high rates of skin cancer because of all the sun exposure...Squamous cell and basal cell carcinoma are really common and while they are not generally lethal they can be really disfiguring...

Moffit Cancer Center's Thomas Sellers, Ph.D. adds, "It is unfortunate that we glamorize a great tan - especially with tanning salons we see increasing rates of melanoma among teenagers."

Many people do not realize that protection from ultraviolet radiation is important year round, even on cloudy days and days in the winter. Francis Marion University's Erin Eaton, Ph.D. points out that, "Even on a cloudy day you get UV radiation…you can also get sun-burned on a winter day which might even be worse because you get the reflection off the snow." In addition, if it's 70 degrees one day and 90 degrees the next, the risk of excessive UV exposure is the same. Dr. Eaton notes that, "Heat doesn't have anything to do with it."

As with many other cancers, the question of how much "dose" of sun one can safely tolerate varies from person to person. Stanford University's Alice Whittemore, Ph.D. says, "Sitting too long in the sun can give people skin cancer. Exposure to sunlight for some people is more dangerous than for others because of genetic reasons." University of California, Davis' Marc Schenker, M.D., M.P.H. adds, "If you are a very fair skinned person, you are at much greater risk of a getting skin induced skin cancer than if you have darker skin."

Taking some relatively simple steps can protect people from skin cancer. The Cleveland Clinic's Dale Shepard, M.D., Ph.D. says, "Melanomas are one of those things that with proper sunscreens, we should actually be having fewer and fewer patients." University of Memphis' James Gurney, Ph.D. agrees noting, "Smart skin protection is important by trying to minimize unnecessary exposure to the sun…If you have the right type of sunblock and you use it effectively, then conventional wisdom is, yes, they are effective." Dr. Eaton suggests, "Avoid tanning booths and use sunscreen… such as SPF 30 and reapply it regularly - at least every few hours."

Late morning and early afternoon hours are the most hazardous for UV exposure outdoors in the continental United States. The National Center for Disease Control recommendations for avoiding excessive UV exposure are:

- Stay in the shade especially during midday hours
- Wear clothing that covers your arms and legs
- Wear a hat with a wide brim to shade your face, head, ears and neck
- Wear sunglasses that wrap around that block both UVA and UVB rays
- Use sunscreen with the sun protective factor (SPF) of 15 or higher with both UVA and UVB protection
- Avoid indoor tanning

Avoid Unnecessary Medical Radiation

The President's Cancer panel has suggested that physicians and patients be much more proactive in reducing unnecessary x-ray procedures such as routine x-rays, nuclear medicine tests, CT scans, fluoroscopy and others. Radiation exposure due to medical imaging poses a cancer risk since it is well-established that radiation damages DNA. Christine Curran, Ph.D., Assistant Professor of Biology at Northern Kentucky University says, "With medical imaging, we have so many scans that we do and we are living longer but there is a question you can ask, 'Do I really need this? Is there a different way? What is the dose of radiation for this?' because we know radiation will damage DNA." Many observers believe that medical and dental radiation is used excessively. LSU's Edward Trapido, Ph.D. concurs adding, "Try not to have unnecessary exposure to radiation. It's not unreasonable to ask when someone goes to a dentist or physician, 'Do I really need to have this x-ray? Do I really need to have this additional scan?'...There is probably overuse of radiation in the medical community."

The President's Cancer Panel recommends that referring physicians be responsible for discussing with the patient the balance between risk and benefit associated with each imaging or nuclear medicine procedure being recommended. Robert Hiatt M.D., Ph.D., Chair, Department of Epidemiology at the University of California,

San Francisco says, "Unnecessary diagnostic radiation is also some-thing individuals should be aware of - talk to your doctor about any CT scan or other types of x-rays that have been proposed and ask if it's really necessary because...you are concerned about the possible contribution to cancer." The President's Cancer Panel also recommended that the effective radiation dose of all imaging and nuclear medicine tests performed should be a required element in patient records and patients should be assisted to reconstruct an estimate of the total medical radiation dose they have received, i.e. their lifetime dose.

Young children are particularly at risk from medical imaging which should be used as sparingly as possible using the lowest dose technology available. University of South Carolina's Anthony Alberg, Ph.D., M.P.H. cautions, "With children, be prudent about the use of radiation." University of Iowa's Bill Fields, Ph.D., M.S. says, "Kids are more radiosensitive at a younger age...One of the cancer risks we have to be attuned to is radiation and kids - like the overuse of CT scans...". Parents and their children's pediatricians need to be proactive on behalf of their children and young patients respectively in this regard. Charnita Zeigler-Johnson, Ph.D., M.P.H., Professor of Cancer Epidemiology at Thomas Jefferson University says, "As children develop, they are at higher risk for certain impacts and you need to keep them away from radiation, for example, everything in moderation but children especially."

Practice Safe Sex and Don't Share Needles

In the earlier review of the Hepatitis and HPV viruses and their vaccines, it was noted that the vaccines are only effective before an infection takes place. That makes prevention an important strategy by taking precautionary measures to avoid these viruses of which many people are still unaware. University of Louisiana's Melinda Oberleitner, R.N., D.N.S. says, "People don't often think about the role that viruses play in causing cancer. We perhaps need to do a better job at getting the word out about sexually transmitted infections that can lead to HPV and Hepatitis B and some of the others." Sharing needles with an infected drug user can lead to HIV, as well as Hepatitis B and Hepatitis C which can increase the risk of liver cancer. In addition, failure to practice safe sex can increase cancer risk. Dr. Marc Schenker says, "Sexually transmitted diseases can be associated with cancer." One can practice safe sex by using a condom and limiting the number of sexual partners. Experts say that the more sexual partners you have in your lifetime, the more likely you are to contract a sexually transmitted infection such as HIV or HPV. People who have HIV or AIDS have a higher risk of cancer of the anus, cervix, lung and immune system. HPV is associated with cervical cancer but it may also increase the risk of cancer of the anus, penis, throat, vulva and vagina.

Caution for Night Shift Workers

Research in recent decades points to the need for real awareness on the part of night shift workers pertaining to increased cancer risk. The first report of an association of exposure to light at night and the risk of breast cancer was in 1987. Since that time, most studies – 17 out of 19, have found such an association. Yong Zhu, Ph.D., Associate Professor at Yale University School of Public Health explains the health risk about working night shifts saying:

> This is against our natural circadian rhythm...which causes circadian disruption...a number of epidemiological studies show that people exposed to light at night such as night shift hospital workers, flight attendants, airline pilots, police officers, have a 50% higher breast cancer risk than day shift workers...and prostate cancer risk in men also increased...

Dr. Zhu elaborates further noting that up until 150 years ago, we only had natural light so most human activities took place during the daylight hours. People slept at night which Dr. Zhu says is probably our evolutionary adaptation to the rotation of the earth. Today, with the advent of electric lights and ample electricity generation, combined with modern society that goes 24-7, we have many night shift workers – approximately 15% of all US workers. The increased cancer risk does not affect all night workers and Dr. Zhu suggests that some people can adapt to the rotating shift work very easily which is probably a result of our genetic makeup. He also noted that blind people did not experience the increased cancer risk as they cannot differentiate night from day and are following their own internal circadian rhythm. Dr. Zhu said it would benefit society if we could at some point identify through genetic analysis what people are best suited for night work. Health experts suggest that night workers follow other recommendations for good health that lower cancer risk such as a nutritious diet, exercise and drinking only moderate amounts of alcohol.

Poverty, Low Education & Cancer Risk

Poverty and low education are also risk factors for cancer. Many public health experts say that the best predictor of poor health is poverty – especially true when combined with low education which is often the case. Americans of lower socioeconomic status (SES): have fewer resources to implement cancer prevention strategies; often have no health insurance with which to pay for cancer screenings; have less knowledge of effective cancer prevention strategies; and, as a result, have a higher incidence of cancer than higher SES individuals. A number of important cancer risks such as smoking, poor nutrition and obesity are much higher in low socioeconomic households. First of all, education matters because it equips people with the knowledge required to implement sound cancer prevention and healthy living strategies. University of Hawaii's Pebbles Fagan, Ph.D., M.P.H. says, "People with higher levels of education are more likely to be physically active, have lower rates of smoking and lower rates of obesity." University of Kentucky's Thomas Tucker, Ph.D. adds:

The real culprits in this are illiteracy and poverty. If you look at smoking rates and lung cancer incidence rates...the high income, high education people have very low rates of both smoking and lung cancer. The low income, low education people have extraordinarily high rates. If we can help people with issues of literacy and poverty, we can then begin to address the issues of cigarette smoking.

Second, having money is helpful in order to implement effective cancer prevention strategies whether it's the ability to buy the best health insurance, a gym membership, organic food, etc. Steven Barger, Ph.D., Professor of Psychology at Northern Arizona University says, "People who have more access to resources are better at managing the manageable threats in their environment." Kurt Ribisl, Ph.D., Professor of Behavioral Health at the University of North Carolina, Chapel Hill says, "Smoking over this century went from being a wealthy person's behavior to one that's now predominantly lower income population." Harvard University's Walter Willet, M.D., Dr. P.H. adds, "If you are poor, you may live in an environment where healthy food is much less available and you don't have transportation to get the healthy food...Among Americans who have incomes below 130% of the federal poverty line, zero percent met all the national dietary goals." David Just, Ph.D., Director of the Cornell Center for Behavioral Economics for Child Nutrition Programs says, "There are these disparities due to income...There are such things as food deserts...".

Lorraine Reitzel, Ph.D., Professor of Psychology at the University of Iowa counters that while knowledge and education are essential, sometimes people have the knowledge and do the wrong things anyway saying:

Most people know by now that smoking causes cancer and is really, really bad for you. Most people don't engage in smoking because they lack the education to know or understand that they can one day die from this. So, in smoking, I don't think education will impact people engaging in unhealthy behaviors. But, I think people of lower socioeconomic status have higher levels of stress, greater levels of financial strain, have fewer resources to, for example, buy nicotine replacement or get smoking cessation counseling...People with higher socioeconomic status, they were able to quit...People who are still smoking is becoming increasingly concentrated within individuals of lower socioeconomic status...A lot of things centered around your socioeconomic status are working against you.,.in some cases it may be tied to lack of education but I think it's a little more tied to income...

David Just, Ph.D., Director of the Cornell Center for Behavioral Economics for Child Nutrition Programs adds:

Low income families feel fresh herbs and vegetables are a huge advantage over canned and frozen fruit and vegetables...which are really cheap and really available at lower incomes but because of that stigma that attached to them, it keeps them artificially from eating healthier... Food that is frozen quickly after it is harvested a lot of times will have more nutrients than the supposed fresh that probably took a week in transit. In canned, there's a little bit of a nutrition difference but it's still better than not having fruits and vegetables in their diet.

Charnita Zeigler-Johnson, Ph.D., M.P.H., Professor of Cancer Epidemiology at Thomas Jefferson University elaborates as to why people with lower education and income struggle:

[Low socioeconomic] people are more at risk for a number of reasons. Some of it is awareness, being aware of what needs to be done or what can be done to reduce their risk.

The other part of it is the resources for those individuals are very different so we have to work at a public or societal level to make a difference in those communities where they have high risk and can do very little on their own to make a difference. We are still working on the best methods to reach those individuals and to actually have them be able to modify their lifestyles...For some who are low income and have low education, they may not realize that those are things that they should do and don't necessarily understand how it relates to certain diseases, such as cancer...One of the most important things that they could do is to establish a relationship with a physician and see him/her regularly.

University of Massachusetts' Laura Vanderberg, Ph.D. adds:

What do people do to change their risk factors? Those are only going to be feasible if you have the means. What if I told you, you could reduce your chances of getting cancer but you can only eat organic foods. Well, that shuts off that level of prevention for a huge population in the US and we have to ask ourselves, and I ask myself all the time, it's not whether or not that's feasible, it's whether or not that's equitable. If cancer prevention is something that only the wealthy can afford, are we as a society okay with that? I personally am not.

Undoubtedly, people with more income and opportunities can more easily understand and implement cancer prevention strategies. However, sometimes the problem is more of lack of knowledge rather than lack of income. Educating people in lower socioeconomic brackets can make a difference such as how to economically buy nutritious food. While many low income people think that they cannot afford to buy healthy food, that is not necessarily true. Yale Cancer Center's Maura Harrigan, M.S., R.D. explains:

Actually, a healthy diet is less expensive. You should reduce your meat consumption. When moving to a predominantly plant-based diet you are reducing your meat purchases, which is a big ticket item. Reduce your purchasing of highly processed foods which are expensive. When you simplify and go to simple, healthy eating it's actually quite economical...I tell patients I can actually reduce your food budget and increase the nutrient content of your family eating, let me show you how to do it.

Jay Thomas Sutliffe, Ph.D., Associate Professor of Public Health at Northern Arizona University concurs adding:

From a nutrition standpoint, when people transition to a plant-based diet, that is actually a money savings. The most expensive items in your cart if you go shopping at the general grocery store are going to be the animal protein products... If a person is going to eat a plant-based diet, eat beans and rice, fruits and vegetables, in the end, you are going to save money. You don't have to be affluent to eat the type of diet that I recommend...

People can also help themselves to afford nutritious food by cutting out a lot of the unhealthy items they purchase such as cigarettes, sodas, potato chips, ice cream, cakes, cookies, and candy that not only get in the way of them buying healthier foods, but are contributing to the high level of overweight and obese people who have low income and low levels of education.

As a society, our failure to do a better job educating low income populations about cancer risks, healthy living, wellness and prevention keeps them at a serious disadvantage. Carlos Crespo, Ph.D., Professor of Community Health at Portland State University sounds a similar theme adding:

We increase exposures in populations who do not know how to protect themselves such as exposure to fat food, exposure to pollution, and by the time these people realize they are getting sick, it is too late. That is morally wrong and financially we cannot afford to do that because we need everybody to be on board and be healthy so everybody benefits...It's expensive to treat sick people. No one is actually thinking about the impact of health inequalities and overall health of the population.

Many people do not understand the opportunities for cancer prevention but that applies even more to people of low education. Louisiana State University's Melinda Sothern, Ph.D. points out that, "When we are educating our patients concerning risk for disease, most of them believe that they inherit disease - that they are pre-ordained to get different diseases. I am convinced that they do not understand the power they have to lower their risk." University of Oklahoma's Mark Doescher, M.D. explains:

Certainly poverty, if you look across cultures, or within the United States, if you look within racial and ethnic groups, poverty is a marker for a host of adverse health outcomes... In the US, the types of food that are the lowest cost per calorie tend to be foods that are not fresh vegetables or higher-quality foods but rather a lot of starch, a lot of corn syrup...The range of foods that you can to afford if you're poor are less and are sometimes not available in neighborhoods where people are poor. Poverty is a marker for other unhealthy behaviors like tobacco use - part which may have to do with marketing and part where you are in life...If you don't have a job, there are higher stress levels and more uncertainty so there's just a host of things that affect people who are at the lower incomes that lead to unhealthy lifestyles and lead to worse health outcomes...Education also matters, it matters a lot...I think education is beneficial, independent to some extent, of income in terms of health outcomes. So, if we improve education as a society, particularly for high need groups, we might do better from a health perspective is a pretty compelling argument...People need to be clamoring for a good education for their children. That happens, but it is much more likely to happen in affluent households...access to the health care system is also an issue for low income populations.

Indeed, in addition to disparities in cancer prevention opportunities between high and low socioeconomic individuals in America, there also is a disparity in the caliber of cancer treatment after it is diagnosed often because of health insurance or lack thereof. University of Arizona's Peter Lance, M.D. explains:

We want our children to get their childhood vaccines, we want them from an early age to have a healthy diet, we want them to read at the right age, we want them to graduate from high school, and as many as possible we want them to go on to further education - the reason I am saying all of those things because the members of our society that that don't make those benchmarks, we know that they don't live as long and they have higher rates for many of the chronic diseases...The thing that is unpalatable is many of the generally accepted metrics or measures of infant mortality, life expectancy, etc., the US does not compare very favorably to other developed countries. If you have good health care and you get diagnosed at the right time, then you have the best outlook of anywhere in the world if you are in the US and you get your cancer treated according to state-of-the-art, state of the science. The gap is between what's available to those who have that access and those who do not in this society and that gap is actually a lot bigger in this society than in many developing countries...Nobody's going to argue if you say, the best care that is available to man or woman is available here in the US and it matches or exceeds anything that's available anywhere else, nobody's going to disagree with that. But is that care getting delivered to the largest number of people? The answer is no.

While the Affordable Care Act, aka ObamaCare, will help reduce the cancer treatment disparities in the US in half of the states that expanded Medicaid eligibility, the other half of the states will continue to have the same treatment disparities as before the law passed. A study at Harvard University Medical School concluded that 45,000 Americans die every year because of lack of health insurance. As a nation, we need to work hard to close the gaps that exist pertaining to opportunities for healthy living as well as cancer prevention and treatment.

While we are fortunate to live in a society that has safety net programs, the government needs to be more effective in administering them so that recipients do not become less healthy as a result of using them. Poorly designed government programs can contribute to obesity. Bruce Ames, Ph.D., Professor Emeritus of Nutrition and Metabolism at the University of California, Berkeley says:

> [Dr. Walter] Willet, who is the best epidemiologist in the country, in the world probably, he told me that the SNAP program [Supplemental Nutrition Assistance Program, a.k.a. food stamps] gets people fatter. That's the big fortification program. They let people buy whatever they want and they buy empty calories whereas in the WIC program [Women, Infant and Children] they are not allowed to buy junk food, they have to buy healthy food and then they get better.

As a nation we need to develop national, state and local strategies to assist our fellow citizens from low socioeconomic backgrounds with programs such as: pre-K education; improved health and physical education; Head Start programs; improved school and technical job training opportunities; healthy communities that address "food deserts"; safe areas to walk and get exercise; mandatory parenting classes in high school; and, providing children with good role models. The fastest way to address at least some of the cancer disparities in the US would be for the half of the states that chose not to expand Medicaid under the Affordable Care Act to join the other half of states that did. That would immediately provide millions of low-income Americans with health insurance who do not have it today which would provide them access to cancer screening tests to get their cancers detected early and properly treated. As described above, early cancer detection can make all the difference in a patient's prognosis. Expanding Medicaid in the half of the states that have not done so yet would make a huge difference in their cancer related outcomes, as well as for proper treatment of many other diseases, and would give them a reasonable shot at living a longer life as is the case with Americans who have health insurance.

Section III

How to Change Your Behavior to Reduce Your Cancer Risk & Protecting our Children

8

How to Change Your Behavior:

Modifying Your Lifestyle to Reduce

Your Risk of Cancer

Let's face it - change is hard and it takes self-discipline to avoid all of the fattening delicious food, avoid excessive alcohol, take the steps needed to drink distilled or filtered water, exercise on a daily basis and go to best grocery store available to buy organic foods. But the reality is, that is what it is going to take for you to get healthy or stay healthy and reduce your cancer risk. Melinda Irwin, Ph.D., Associate Professor of Chronic Disease Epidemiology and Co-Director of the Cancer Prevention and Control Program at Yale University succinctly states, "Behavior change is extremely difficult." As important as public policy is, individuals must take control of their own destiny, to the extent their circumstances permit, to strive to modify their behaviors that impact their health. This very much needs to occur at a conscious level which requires that one be ever vigilant in order to resist the bombardment of advertising for unhealthy products, cultural norms, and fad diets - all of which requires that you, as an individual, take steps to strengthen self-discipline in an environment that is all too often hostile to healthy living. As you develop good habits, it will become easier but that's not to say it will ever be easy. What's easy is to be lazy, give in to all of the temptations and totally lose control of your health. University of Texas Medical School's Robert Amato, D.O. says about self-control, "I am very health oriented. I work out every day. But it's a discipline that you have to develop and once you develop the habit, it becomes a natural thing to do."

Even if you are moving forward according to your plan, there will be times when you relapse into the old bad habits, but that is natural and it happens to everybody – nobody is perfect. However, if you are really committed to a life of healthy living for you and your family, you will work hard to stay with it. Patrick Bordnick, Ph.D., Associate Professor at the Graduate College of Social Work at the University of Houston and Director of their Center for Drug and Policy Research says:

> Cues in our environment trigger memories and feelings of wanting which help trigger relapses...and increase our cravings for alcohol, cigarettes, and food...Research shows that if you put people in a bar, it increases their craving for alcohol and cigarettes...As a behaviorist, I think you can develop those skills but every day can be a challenge. It's not super difficult to figure out how to get someone off drugs, or to lose weight – it is keeping them from relapsing and gaining that weight back or, if it is an addiction, from relapsing to become a smoker or drinker again...What it comes down to is making changes across your life - cognitive, behavioral, potentially environmental changes - there's a lot that goes into it...Most people gain the weight back after losing it because they never made all of these changes.

Yale Cancer Center's Maura Harrigan, M.S., R.D. says, "Our focus has to be on establishing healthy routines and being able to sustain them." It takes a lot of self-discipline or self-control to make hard choices and to stick with them so you should work hard on this aspect of your life. You should start with small changes and then gradually work your way up step-by-step, creating good habits and improving self-discipline along the way. For example, if you are starting an exercise program, start small by taking the stairs instead of the elevator, for example, or walk around the block where you live. Roy Baumeister, Ph.D., Professor of Psychology at Florida State University and Author of the New York Times Best Seller, "Willpower: Rediscovering the Greatest Human Strength" says:

> What we find is self-control is like a muscle. When you exercise it regularly, it gets stronger… So the first thing to do is strengthen the self-control 'muscle' - start small by walking to get a little exercise, making your bed, making small improvements in yourself, etc…Small changes over a long period of time will build into long-term positive effects….to be the person that you want to be.

You must be confident that you can make lifestyle changes. Having confidence in your ability to make the change will increase your likelihood of success. Minimizing temptations is also important. If you know you eat too many sweets or drink too much alcohol, for example, your self-discipline should start in the grocery store by not buying them.

Making a Commitment to Change

Making a commitment to a lifelong change to live healthy and to reduce your risk of cancer and other diseases is a big deal and a big change for most people. As part of your preparation for this most positive change in your life, consider making a written commitment, or pledge to yourself, that you will work diligently to meet your new lifetime goal of healthy living. Place it in a prominent but private place and look at it regularly. Consider attaching to this document a picture of someone you know and love – you are doing this not only for yourself but the people in your life who would like to see you around for awhile. The pledge might go something like this:

My Pledge to Myself

I hereby pledge to do my very best to adhere to my specific goals for healthy living and lifestyle changes by following the steps below as consistently as possible in order to improve my health, feel better and reduce my risk of cancer, heart disease, diabetes and other diseases. I recognize that change is very hard for most people and even in doing my best, there will be times when I will not meet these goals and that I am not unusual in this regard. Those minor setbacks will not prevent me from doing my best to honor my long-term commitment to these principles of good health.

Regardless of how I fare in this regard, I also promise to value myself because I am a good, unique and beautiful person who will not be defined by this alone or what others think of me. I will begin this important change in my life by carefully reading each of the steps below and apply the lessons that I have learned and will continue to learn about healthy living so that I fully understand what I have to do and why I am doing it. I will post this pledge and the steps described below in a prominent location so that I can review them regularly so I do not forget my pledge or to take all of the steps necessary in fulfilling it.

I acknowledge that achieving good physical, mental and emotional health involves many variables such as environment, genetics and medical care. However, personal lifestyle choices have been proven indisputably to be one of the most important determinants of good health.

Therefore, I believe that following the steps below as consistently as I possibly can will help maximize my chances of being healthy which, if achieved, may allow me to spend many years doing the things that I enjoy in life with those who I care about the most.

Steps to Good Health – My Checklist

1. Make the pledge above – read it frequently along with these steps
2. Get ready - change is hard
3. Eat a nutritious, well-balanced diet and as much organic food as possible – take a good multi-vitamin/mineral daily
4. Watch my weight and check it frequently
5. Drink steamed distilled or filtered water and cut out the soft drinks
6. Exercise almost every day
7. Get at least 7 to 8 hours sleep a night
8. Live as safely as possible such as avoiding exposure to synthetic environmental chemicals and other carcinogens, safe driving, etc.
9. Perform self-exams and get my cancer screenings such as mammography, colonoscopy, PAP smears and PSA – talk to my doctor about what screening tests apply to me
10. Talk to my doctor about me and my kids getting vaccinated against Hepatitis B and HPV viruses
11. See my primary care physician regularly and mental health professional, as needed
12. Manage my chronic medical condition such as cancer, heart disease or diabetes, if any
13. Limit alcohol consumption and avoid illegal drugs
14. Avoid air pollution as much as possible and install the best possible air filter my home
15. Use sunscreen with the sun protective factor (SPF) of 15 or higher with both UVA and UVB protection
16. Quit smoking, if applicable, or never start
17. Brush my teeth at least 2x per day, floss daily and see a dentist every 6 months or annually
18. Develop my mind - commit to lifelong learning

19. Avoid miscellaneous risks such as minimizing night shifts and late hours; practicing safe sex; testing my home for radon; and, avoiding excessive medical radiation
20. Seek help and support as needed from a friend, family member, counselor, therapist or wellness coach

All of the steps above will be needed to attain and then maintain good health. Most are directly related to a sound cancer prevention program and will also help to prevent other diseases since a number of major diseases share common risk factors. For example, as mentioned earlier, a poor diet, lack of exercise, overweight and obesity are well-established risk factors for three of the biggest diseases in America – cancer, heart disease and diabetes. Also, realize that you are not alone. Everyone needs a little support, especially when making a big change. Robert Amato, D.O., Professor of Oncology at the University of Texas Medical School and Chief of the Division of Oncology at Memorial Hermann Cancer Center says:

> If a husband and wife are not participating together in a dietary change, it will be an enormous challenge. The thing that I hear commonly is, 'We are doing it as a family'. And those people are more successful at it because now they are meeting with the nutritionist at the Cancer Center and evolving into a family plan of diet rather than one individual person's diet and now they don't have to cook two separate meals, or have two separate refrigerators, they are now doing it as a family. Family buy-in, it works.

Joel Hughes, Ph.D., Professor of Psychology at Kent State University adds:

> Social support is very important as are positive messages. Give positive messages like 'I really appreciate what you're trying to do' or 'I know this is going to be really hard'. When the people making a lifestyle change get irritable which

most people do when they stop smoking, for example, say 'I'm going to give you a break'...We have template letters that we would have people write to their support people explaining some of the things they were likely to see - I am going to be stressed out, there is a chance I will have a slip up, please don't punish me.

So, if needed, talk to a family member, wellness coach, your doctor or a trusted friend or relative. They can help keep you get on track or get you back on track. Finally, do not be too hard on yourself, set realistic goals and don't give up! Almost everyone who tries to change will experience some setbacks. Remember, this is a marathon and not a sprint. To be successful, you have to commit to a lifetime change.

9

Protecting our Children

Pregnant Mothers, Fetuses, Babies, Children and Environmental Exposures

Cancer experts say that fetuses, babies, children and adolescents all need very special attention because their tissues are developing so rapidly which makes them even more susceptible to the cancer risks from environmental exposures than adults. Cindy Battie, Ph.D., Professor of Public Health at the University of North Florida says, "What we should be considering is our children. That earlier onset of cancer, that is a problem...the childhood cancers." It's not just environmental exposures that need to be avoided but rather a whole series of healthy behaviors need to be embarked on because public health experts agree that healthy habits started early in life lay the foundations for a lifetime of healthy living and good health. While we cannot change our past, we can all pledge from this point forward to do better for ourselves and our children, the latter who we want to start off on the right footing as early as possible. Laura Vanderberg, Ph.D., Professor of Environmental Health at University of Massachusetts School of Public Health Sciences says:

> Unfortunately, all of that dairy that I consumed as a child was filled with organic pollutants and are now stored inside my body. So, I am essentially a little depot. As I get pregnant, as I breast-feed, I will be giving those pollutants to my offspring. The choices that I made when I was 10 years old, I

have to pay for the next 20, 30 years because of how long these chemicals persist in bodies. That seems like an unfair burden for a 10-year-old...We have to put the burden of avoidance on the right people and we have a right to know what's in the products we buy at the store.

Fetuses, infants and young children are particularly susceptible to toxic chemicals including carcinogens due to rapid tissue development and cell division that occurs at a young age. Even toxins that a mother is exposed to can lead to childhood cancers. Yawei Zhang, M.D., Ph.D. M.P.H., Associate Professor of Cancer Epidemiology at the Yale School of Medicine says, "Right now there is a hypotheses that many diseases that occur in adulthood have their origins in fetal life." Rashmi Kaul, Ph.D., Associate Professor of Immunology at Oklahoma State University says, "Everything is determined when the baby is being made and the genes are being affected...The first trimester is a very, very sensitive time when tissues and vital organs are developing rapidly...". Pregnant women and those considering having children must be ever vigilant about all of their health habits and what they do to their bodies as it can affect their unborn babies or those not yet conceived.

As noted earlier, there is solid evidence of environmental chemicals being passed on from mothers to their unborn babies. University of Kentucky's Susan Arnold, M.D. says of the American Academy of Pediatrics statement that babies in America are born 'pre-polluted':

> To me, that is a tragedy because having been a mother and being a mother, the most important thing to me was protecting my children, and my children, probably like other children, came out exposed. They were exposed to toxins before they even had a choice and that's because of the lack of knowledge about the toxins that we are exposed to.

It's possible that early exposures to toxic chemicals very early in life may be contributing to some childhood cancers as well as those that are appearing later in life. University of Pittsburgh's Thomas Kensler, Ph.D. notes that the latency period or time to develop cancer in fetuses may "occur more quickly because many of the cells are replicating and that's when they're most vulnerable to attack by carcinogens." Linda Birnbaum, Ph.D., Director of the National Institute of Environmental Health Science adds:

> Before birth and during infancy are very vulnerable times... puberty is a very vulnerable time and pregnancy is a vulnerable time for the mother as well as the developing fetus... Those are times that we have even more opportunities for prevention to occur...If a woman smokes when she's pregnant, her offspring are much more likely to be obese, not necessarily when they're born...but by the age of 10 and it persists throughout adulthood. They tend to be at more risk of obesity...We are seeing cancers in children which obviously isn't something that we used to think much about... There is data now showing associations between different kinds of environmental exposures and certain kinds of childhood cancers.

Laura Anderko, Ph.D., R.N. Cancer Epidemiologist and Fellow at the Center for Social Justice at Georgetown University concurs saying, "If your mom smoked when she was pregnant with you, you are three times more likely of being born with a learning disability. [Drugs] that moms took during pregnancies to prevent miscarriages - their daughters have all sorts of reproductive cancers as a result. Fetuses and kids are particularly susceptible due to these windows of vulnerability." Alice Whittemore, Ph.D., Professor of Health Policy, Epidemiology and Biostatistics at Stanford University agrees explaining:

> Women who smoke during pregnancy have babies with lower birth weight and have more problems and of course

there is fetal alcohol syndrome. Women who drink excessively while pregnant, they can cause lifetime medical and
mental disorders on the part of the children...the in utero
fetus is very vulnerable to exposures like radiation, tobacco
and alcohol.

Michael Skinner, Ph.D., Professor of Biochemistry at Washington
State University elaborates on these most important developmen-
tal periods saying:

> When an organ starts to develop, in its early stages, this is
> a critical time for an environmental exposure, to shift how
> those cells function from then and later in life. For mammary
> glands, for example, for breast cancer, the time the mam-
> mary gland is rapidly developing initially is during the early
> stages of puberty. So when a young teenage girl is exposed
> to something like BPAs in plastics at high levels for a couple
> of years, she is changing her epigenetic programming, those
> chemical modifications to DNA in her mammary epithelial
> cells. That then will shift, from then on and later in life what
> genes are 'on' and 'off'. Therefore, the mammary epithelial
> cells has a shifted gene expression profile in terms of what
> genes are on or off. And then later in life, that shift, when
> you're in your 40s or 50s will lead to the susceptibility to
> then develop a transformed tumor development in terms
> of mammary glands - breast cancer. So the origins of the
> disease wasn't what was going on in your 40s or 50s but
> probably more what was going on when you were in puberty
> so that is what's called a direct exposure epigenetic effect
> influencing the individual exposed...The concept of the
> 'Developmental Origins of Disease' which has been around
> for 15 or 20 years, basically says early life exposures within
> the individual and tissues is really what is the causal factor in
> later life for disease onset... Whatever you do during preg-
> nancy will have more of an impact on the disease of your

children than anything else. If you want to have an impact on the disease of your children, you have to be super cautious about what you're exposed to during pregnancy. Then, the next step is, those children postnatal are also very sensitive so preventing those children's exposures is also important and then during puberty, particularly for breast and prostate, is the most critical time to deal with it...So even though our environment is contaminated, we can actually move towards, at least in those critical times of development, trying to keep our children from those levels of exposure when they are most critical.

The Siteman Cancer Center's Graham Coditz, M.D., Dr. P.H. illustrates the point with a lesson from history saying, "Young people are more at risk. The classic example is the atomic bomb dropped on Hiroshima at the end of the Second World War. The women who were under 20 at the time the bomb was dropped had substantial higher risk of breast cancer than the women who were older."

Fighting Childhood Obesity

With one of six children in American being obese, we really will have to work hard to turn this trend around but there is hope. Susan Mayne, Ph.D., Professor of Epidemiology and Associate Director of the Yale Cancer Center explains:

Progress is being made. For the first time, we are now seeing declines in childhood obesity in certain parts of the country and we turned around trends that were going up, going up, going up. So, it is possible to impact it. From a cancer prevention point of view, it's one of the most important things we can do.

John Erdman, Ph.D., Professor of Food Science and Human Nutrition at the University of Illinois adds, "Getting a good start on the right diet early in life makes a big difference in terms of prevalence [of cancer] later on." Prospective parents as well as new parents should take heed of the problem and the pitfalls that beset so many parents of the past, often because of lack of knowledge about the right things to do. Jamie Ard, M.D., Co-director of the Weight Management Center at Wake Forest Baptist Medical Center explains:

> We are learning that early in the development of a child, even from conception, that the influence of what the mother is doing and what the parents are doing collectively is programming that child and that programming is genetic as well as behavioral and psychological…Even the amount of weight that the mother gains during pregnancy, we are learning, has influence on the size of the infant and the toddler's risk of being overweight in the first few years of life.

Joshua Muscat, Ph.D., an Epidemiologist and Professor of Health Science at the Penn State Cancer Institute says about the fight against childhood obesity:

> It's early education for kids. It really starts with kids learning healthy habits in childhood so the issue for society is that we try to prevent this in the future, the best way to do this is to try to maintain healthy dietary habits in children so that they won't adopt these unhealthy lifestyle habits as adults. Once the [unhealthy habits] are started, it's very difficult to change that…The best thing we can do in terms of cancer prevention and disease prevention in the future, is to provide nutritious foods to children, foods that are low in calories and high in nutrients and low in fats and carbohydrates and once they learn how to eat those types of diets, then they can carry those dietary habits into the future.

Peter Lance, M.D., Professor of Medicine, Molecular and Cellular Biology and Public Health and Chief Cancer Prevention and Control Officer at the University of Arizona adds that children:

> ...are not taking enough physical activity. We are really lacking and where we really need progress is in the behavioral sciences. To begin to understand what things works that will make sure kids from an early age get plenty of exercise... What are the simple effective ways that we can actually inculcate into the population the elements of healthy lifestyles. In the end, that's where we have to go if we want a population to change and that's what we are talking about. Obesity and lack of physical activity are important risk factors for the major cancers...

All public health experts agree that the foundations for good health are laid very early in life. For this to happen, parents must be good role models for their children. James Gurney, Ph.D., Professor of Epidemiology at the University of Memphis School of Public Health explains:

> There is evidence now to show that the mechanisms that lead to obesity are laid down pretty early in life and most of us are not able to make dramatic behavioral changes and weight is not easy to lose. With obesity, I think we really need to be thinking about preventative measures. Developing a culture within young families of raising their children in such a way to minimize the risk of excess weight and things associated with it like sugary drinks, lack of exercise, high degree of screen time like television and whatnot, the size of our meals, the types of food that we eat, we tend to eat salty, fatty, sugary foods and all of that lends itself to putting on weight...School systems have cut physical activity programs although I know there are efforts now to try to increase that in many ways...Most kids are being very, very strongly

influenced by their parents and so the message has to be directed to the parents, they have to buy-in and implement it at a relatively young age for us to hope to really see this thing turn around.

University of Louisiana's Melinda Oberleitner, R.N., D.N.S. adds:

Obesity starts as early as childhood and the behaviors and the foods that we become accustomed to eating as we are growing up when we really do not have control over what we are eating because we are getting most of our nutrients from whatever our parents are providing and to break the cycle is very difficult.

Northern Arizona University's Jay Thomas Sutliffe, Ph.D. adds:

I don't see the improvement yet [in our children's diets]. There's a lot of money being spent on childhood obesity, gardens in elementary school. We are doing all these different things and then we get home and the parents grab the food, throw it in the microwave and flop it down on the TV tray and then let the kid play the videogame...I am cautiously optimistic that we are going to make an impact... behavior change is where it's at.

Thomas Tucker, Ph.D., Associate Director of Cancer Prevention of the Markey Cancer Center at the University of Kentucky agrees saying, "More kids are spending time inside playing computer games and less time out exercising."

Parents should start early in their children's lives and not wait too late when the job becomes more difficult. Melinda Sothern, Ph.D., Professor of Behavioral and Community Health Sciences and Exercise Physiologist at Louisiana State University says, "It's very hard to wait until your children are teenagers to start setting healthy living rules." Parents who are trying to change the behavior of children who are overweight or obese will have to work hard to change the behavior and even may have to improve their own parenting skills to be successful. Elena Reyes, Ph.D., Associate Professor and Director of Behavioral Medicine at Florida State University explains:

> What are things that parents might say, 'Well, I would like to learn how to talk to my kids better'...What does that have to do with getting little Johnny to lose weight? Well, for those parents, they really may not have the skills that would allow for them to exchange information with their child about their eating habits and do it in a way that does not produce conflict in the home because every time they tell little Johnny, 'No you can't have another piece of bacon', Johnny throws a fit, says mommy is mean...So the fact that this parent doesn't have a set of behaviors that she can use to try to dialogue with her child and train the child in a way without conflict is an impediment to his losing weight...There is some research out there indicating that the quality of life for children who are obese is equivalent to the quality of life for children with cancer. They are never picked for the team. They are outsiders...

Children spend a good part of their lives in schools and they need to be provided with rigorous physical education, lots of physical activity as well as quality health education programs. Peter Shields, M.D., a medical oncologist and Deputy Director of the James Cancer Center at Ohio State University says, "We need physical education in elementary schools, middle school and high school. If we could get young people into healthy lifestyles, a lifelong lifestyle, getting these kids eating better, that to me makes the most sense." Good eating habits start early and schools have a responsibility to provide nutritious food for children during school hours and educate them about proper nutrition. A good starting point would be assuring that sufficient funding is available for school lunch programs. University of Kentucky's Nancy Schoenberg, Ph.D. explains that, "The school lunch program operates on two dollars per lunch per day. Now, how are you going to be able to have an incredible vegetable rich and palatable school lunch program when you're operating on such a thin financial margins."

As children get a little older with improved reasoning skills, parents should not only model healthy behavior for their children but be willing to explain why it is important. Roy Baumeister, Ph.D., Professor of Psychology at Florida State University says:

> Explain the rules at all times and your reasoning and as the child gets older, like a teenager, can understand the rules in a more complex way and maybe agree to them and understand why they are acceptable and make a personal commitment. That way they get more involved in regulating themselves.

The vast majority of cancer risks described in this book also apply to children who should: avoid unnecessary exposure to environmental chemicals; drink filtered or distilled water; eat organic food and lots of fruits and vegetables; not start smoking; not drink alcohol; get vaccinated against Hepatitis B and HPV; breathe clean air; get adequate sleep; get plenty of exercise; and, as Francis Marion University's Erin Eaton, Ph.D. reminds us, "Protect children against sunburn...".

All of this is not to say that as children get older, they cannot change the course of their lives – it will simply be more difficult for them if they get off to a bad start in life with unhealthy habits and exposures. Walter Willet, M.D., Dr. P.H., Professor of Epidemiology and Nutrition and Chair of the Department of Nutrition at the Harvard School of Public Health explains, "Still, what happens later in life is extremely important and can override some of those [genetic or epigenetic] tendencies."

Section IV

New Developments in Cancer

Treatment & Conclusion

10

Promising Developments
in Cancer Treatment

Screening, Early Detection & Your Primary Care Physician

Before discussing promising cancer treatments on the horizon, it is worth emphasizing what was mentioned in the beginning of this book about the importance of early detection of cancer. That is, early detection and the most successful treatments are often closely related. This is very important as early detection generally improves the prognosis for patients – often substantially. This is also true for cancer survivors who need to be vigilant about the possibility of a cancer returning and to detect it as early as possible. If caught early enough, the cancer can usually be successfully treated before it metastasizes and spreads to the lymph nodes or an organ which makes the prognosis much more problematic?

East Carolina University's Dr. Paul Walker explains:

> The most exciting advance in treating cancer is early detection…[for some cancers] patients diagnosed with screening have a 92% cure so if you have something that could produce a 92% cure rate well, it's not the treatment – it's the early detection…Not having it is best; detecting it early is second because you get a much higher cure with less treatment…

At least that is the closest thing to a "cure" there is with cancer given that once someone has been diagnosed with cancer even with early detection, there is an increased risk of getting cancer again in the future. After cancer treatment, if there is no detectable sign of cancer remaining, the patient is said to have experienced a complete remission. The National Cancer Institute defines complete remission as, "The disappearance of all signs of cancer in response to treatment" and adds "This does not always mean the cancer has been cured." It is possible that for some people after treatment, there are still cancer cells in the body that cannot be detected by any current technology. Gary Meadows, Ph.D., Professor of Pharmaceutical Science at Washington State University explains:

> Total remission is that you cannot detect the cancer. That does not mean there are still not cancer cells in your body. Really, the only way that you can say somebody is cured of cancer is how long they survive…We never really talk about cures with cancer. We talk about long-term survivors because you can never really be sure if you got rid of all of the cancer cells. They can lie dormant in your body and that's okay too and that's another area we are looking at from a research point of view. As long as you can keep cancer cells dormant and suppressed in your body, you can live with cancer.

It is important to keep in mind, however, that early detection of cancer is not just your doctor's job, but is your responsibility as well. In addition to the cancer screenings mentioned above that are performed at medical facilities, self-awareness of any signs of changes in your health and self-examination in the privacy of your own home is a tremendously important part of cancer prevention and early detection. Simply put, being in tune with your own body is essential. Self-awareness and self-examinations will help you to get prompt medical screening procedures and appropriate medical care if you are showing early signs of cancer or precancerous lesions. Examples of self-awareness can be demonstrated in various ways such as an individual who notices a blotch or other skin change or abnormality that could possibly be a sign of early skin cancer. Another is a woman who detects a small lump during a self-breast examination that could possibly be an early sign of breast cancer. A third example could be a man who notices rectal bleeding that could be an early sign of colon cancer. The American Cancer Society recommends that you be on the lookout for the following changes in your health:

- A change in bowel or bladder habits
- A sore throat that does not heal
- Unusual bleeding or discharge
- Thickening or lump in the breast or elsewhere
- Indigestion or difficulty in swallowing
- Obvious change in a wart or mole
- Nagging cough or hoarseness

These and other early warning signs of potential cancer should be reported immediately to your primary care physician. While people hear the term "primary care physician" frequently, as a point of clarification, primary care physicians (PCPs) fall under four categories of physicians as follows:

1. Internists: (not to be confused with interns which is an old term used to describe someone just out of medical school serving his/her first year of residency) - an internist is an Internal Medicine physician who can diagnose and treat a wide range of medical conditions in adults.

2. Family Practitioners (also referred to as Family Medicine physicians): similar to internists described above in that they are well trained to diagnose and treat a wide range of medical conditions but family practitioners are trained to care for both adults and children. There are a smaller number of

physicians often referred to Med-Peds who have achieved separate board certifications in both Internal Medicine and Pediatrics and who also take care of both adults and children.

3. Pediatricians: physicians who care for children of all ages including late teens.

4. OB-GYN (obstetrics/gynecology): provide care to female patients only and specialize in the reproductive system in women. They are sometimes included in the category of primary care since many women get a great deal of their routine care from them.

By reporting early warning signs of a potential cancer to your primary care physician, he or she can immediately order the necessary diagnostic tests such as various laboratory tests and/or imaging exams such as x-rays, CT (computerized axial tomography) scans, or MRI (magnetic resonance imaging). Those diagnostic tests and others will help to confirm or rule out the presence of cancer. It cannot be emphasized enough how important it is for you to be very proactive in your own health and to select a primary care physician who will be your partner in all matters pertaining to your health. Remember, early detection of cancer or precancerous lesions can save your life.

Promising Cancer Treatments on the Horizon

New cancer treatments are constantly being developed so let's hear what some experts say about several major cancer treatment areas and some of the latest thinking about each of those in their own words. It is intended for those who have a particular interest in emerging cancer treatments with a bit of the science behind it and what some of the researchers think in terms of their prospects for success. These treatments include surgery which, for many cancer patients, is the first treatment they encounter in order to remove a tumor, part of an organ, lymph nodes, etc. Next will be remarks from cancer experts about developments in targeted chemotherapy, immunotherapy and radiation therapy. These therapies attempt to increasingly target diseased tissue while protecting as much surrounding healthy tissue as possible which addresses a major problem in cancer treatment. As noted earlier, most of today's chemotherapy also damages healthy tissue and has very serious side effects for patients.

Surgery

Paul Dale, M.D., Chief of Surgical Oncology at the Ellis Fischel Cancer Center and Professor of Medical Research at the University of Missouri School of Medicine describes some of the progress in the area of cancer surgery as follows:

> Surgery is still the mainstay for most cancers. If we can remove your tumor, in general, you will do better than if we cannot remove it. We are doing more surgeries on smaller tumors because they are being detected sooner...One of the most exciting advances that has hit surgical oncology in the last 10 years is the concept of the sentinel node biopsy... The sentinel node biopsy is the concept that cancers of the skin and the breast and even of some other organs drain from the tumor to one lymph node first. That's called the sentinel node like the sentinel guard of a castle who is the first guard to get shot. The sentinel node captures the cancer cells and the theory is before it spreads to other lymph nodes, or throughout the body, it stays in that one sentinel node. If you can identify that sentinel node and take it out, you can determine whether it has or has not spread. Ten years ago, if you had breast cancer, I would have to remove your breast and all of your lymph nodes. Now, I take out one lymph node if there is no cancer in that one lymph node, which is true in 30% of patients. Then you do not have to

have all of your lymph nodes removed and that's a huge advancement in the treatment of melanoma, breast cancer, some other head and neck cancers and other cancers that are being investigated for the sentinel node technique. That technique has really reduced the amount of surgery required for a lot of patients who have cancer...Other techniques include oblation which has come along. For example, nowadays, with non-resectable tumors of the liver...we can burn these with radiofrequency therapy. It's almost to the point where we are microwaving the small tumors in the liver - you can do very tight burns on tumors that are non-resectable in the liver, killing the tumors, letting them turn to scar tissue and leaving the rest of the liver... Direct therapies are becoming more and more popular. I think in the future, we are probably going to have direct therapies where I can actually inject you with a material...that might show where the cancer cells are in your body which will allow us to go and surgically remove just cancer involved lymph nodes...Also, robotic surgery has come a long way...not in every type of cancer but in certain applications, the da Vinci [surgical robotic device] has allowed us to do much quicker and even safer operations such as prostatectomy in males. It's made it much easier to do that dissection in very tight places where you really can't get your hands down to sew, you can get the robotic arms down there...that allows us to operate in very tight fitting places...Minimally invasive types of surgical procedures is where we are going now. From 1900 to the 1970s, radical, radical, radical was the mainstay - radically remove everything. For example, in breast cancer, they didn't just remove the breast but the muscles underneath the breast in the past - but no more. What we are finding now is that you don't have to be quite as radical which is why we can save breasts and not remove them radically anymore...In general, I do think that having surgery in this day and age is a lot better than having it 10, 20 or 30 years ago...Today, the patients are often able to go home the next day and they do outstanding at home and many surgeries are being moved from inpatient to an outpatient basis and patients are certainly benefiting from these advances...We have reduced postoperative infections, postoperative morbidity and postoperative mortality - all are going down because of improved technology, improved techniques, better postoperative care and better ICU care...Whether patients get chemotherapy or radiation therapy after their cancer surgery depends on the stage of the tumor. Broadly speaking, if the tumor was localized and completely removed - no spread to the lymph nodes, then maybe no chemotherapy or radiation is indicated. If the cancer has spread to the lymph nodes, then perhaps chemotherapy or radiation will help that patient to live longer.

John Bell, M.D., a surgical oncologist and Director of the Cancer Institute at the University of Tennessee adds that there have been advances in:

...all of the various forms of minimally invasive surgery including laparoscopic approaches as well as robotic approaches... With many cancers we used to have to do major open surgery which are now often times very safe using a form of minimally invasive surgery that allows the patient to recover and return to a normal life in a much shorter period of time and yet still achieve the same control of their disease that we used to be able to do with large open surgeries...Today, the most common robotic cancer surgeries would be done in female malignancies such as ovarian, uterine, and cervical... there's more experience and longevity in that field of robotic cancer surgery [with those cancers] than any others...

Surgeons can also remove cancerous tissues or suspected cancerous tissue for lab analysis which today can give us more information than ever before. Dean Hosgood, Ph.D., M.P.H., at Albert Einstein College of Medicine explains:

> A surgeon can take a little biopsy of a tumor...[the lab can] extract the DNA of the tumor...and genotype it for the specific characteristics we are looking for in those genes and if those are present, that would dictate what treatment regimen that patient would be put on...would go on to have more targeted treatment...and we see tremendous difference in response...

Dale Shepard, M.D., Ph.D., a medical oncologist with the Cleveland Clinic explains:

> There is some fascinating stuff going on with linking drugs to receptors...By doing that you can have the chemotherapy delivered specifically to the cells that are most likely to need the treatment of that chemotherapy...Genomics is certainly something you hear about. There is no end to the buzz about personalized medicine and looking at genomics in terms of really thinking about not treating tumors by geography because when you think about how we treat cancers now - people specialize in lung cancer or colon cancer or kidney cancer and the treatments that patients get are specific to the organ that is involved...Really, the thought is that there may be a genetic change in those cells that trigger them to become tumors and maybe with those genetic changes there are some common pathways to a lot of different tumors, so maybe we should be moving things more to treating those underlying genomic changes rather than just treating by body area...The problem is there are a lot of genomic changes we know that occur but we don't necessarily have drugs to target them...We know there is a defect there but we don't necessarily know what to do about it. Our ability to design drugs that actually target pathways is lagging but I think is actually

one of the promising areas. I think it gives encouragement to this concept of treating based on genetic or genomic changes. If you think about how we used to develop drugs, we used to just use drugs that kill cells that grew quickly and if you look at traditional chemotherapy agents, you're looking at inhibiting DNA production and cells that grow quickly, get affected more quickly than their neighbors so that you get specificity... In terms of immunotherapies for other tumors, we are still trying to understand what tumors are best suited for that kind of therapy and what agents might be best for those particular diseases.

Howard Gross, M.D., Medical Oncologist with the Dayton Clinical Oncology Program adds:

The targeted chemotherapy where the treatment is targeted to certain molecular changes that is causing the cancer versus some bomb of chemotherapy where you are just trying to prevent cancer cells from dividing. That is certainly were a lot of research and medical oncology is going... Immunotherapy is very exciting and has been going on since the 1970s...There are certainly some exciting things in the works...We are doing a better job treating the whole patient rather than the chemotherapy [team] is going off and doing one thing while ignoring what the surgeons and radiation therapists are doing. It is more of a team effort than it ever has been... since they were able to identify the human genome, I think the genetics and the therapy based on that is where it's going to be in the future.

Gary Meadows, Ph.D., Professor of Pharmaceutical Science at Washington State University says:

There is a lot of money being invested by the pharmaceutical industry in developing more targeted therapies. There's thousands of them that get out on the market for clinical trials each year. A lot of them fail but there have been some successes in targeting various signaling pathways or genes or what have you and again we will have to be using all these combinations because one problem with cancer that is treated with a combination of drugs, whatever that might be, that places a selective pressure on the cancer cell...the cancer is there wanting to survive and it's got all these mutations, the cancer cells have an ability, to ultimately develop resistance to those therapies and so the therapy is only partially effective. In most cases, you can never kill all the cancer cells because the cancer adapts to the selective pressure you are putting on it with the chemotherapy that you are giving the patient...You can only use these therapies once [because the cancer cells develop resistance to them]...With [current] chemotherapy, there is a systemic toxicity. With these more targeted therapies that are targeting a specific molecule, we are finding that they are less toxic. There are approaches now that deliver the more targeted therapies that will select out only the cancer cells and leave the normal cells alone. This is an approach a lot of people are taking about although most of it is still experimental.

The previous paragraph was about targeted chemotherapy but then there is immunotherapy of which Dr. Meadows explains:

What we are trying to do is to activate specific types of immune cells that are known to be able to kill the cancer cells...This has emerged again as another potentially more successful way of treating cancer. Again, it's probably an approach that will need to be combined, it will be a multiple type of targeted approach. Activating the immune system, we know that there are certain cells in the immune system that can kill tumor cells. There are so-called cytotoxic T-cells - they are natural killer cells. One of the problems with previous immunotherapies was trying to get the cells activated and targeted to the tumors. The other problem that we are trying to counteract, is that when you stimulate the immune system - there's good checks and balances on the immune system. You don't want an activated immune system all the time because that would be toxic. So, in the course of activating the immune system, you can also activate cells that are suppressor cells that eventually inactivate those cells that you are activating to kill the tumor cells...One of the roles of the immune system is to get rid of those genetically defective cells...The immune system itself can get overwhelmed...and can decline with age...they do respond to stimulating factors...Exercise and what we eat [a nutritious diet] can help... As the cancer grows or maybe it's in an area that is less accessible to the immune system and the immune system is not seeing those cells readily until they get fluffed off and enter the blood. The first line of defense are natural killer cells. They have an innate ability to bind to a cancer cell and once that binding occurs, there are these granules that are present in the natural killer cells that contain some enzymes and other proteins, these enzymes are released, the proteins are released into the tumor cell that results in the binding and are able to then cause destruction of the tumor cells...The T-cells, the cytotoxic cells, require activation before they can kill...Most of the success right now is in the melanoma field - skin cancer... Melanoma is a horrible disease and it is innately resistant to chemotherapy and other therapeutic approaches. That's where most of the success has been. Some of the immune therapies have been more promising than the chemotherapies [with melanomas]...There still can be some toxicity [to surrounding tissues] and it is individual, everybody is different. Some people won't see much toxicity and some will not be able to take the drug and that's all based on our own individual makeup... There is a lot of research going on in that area to find out

number one, how dormancy is regulated. And it may be possible in the future to develop sort of a maintenance program
for keeping those cells dormant because many times what
kills you mostly from cancer is that it spreads throughout
the body and starts to grow in various organs and that it
compromises the functions of those various organs...[these
new treatment approaches] may take up to five to ten years
– it's a slow process...Targeted therapies, the micro RNA
approaches, and the immunotherapy approaches, I think all
of those we need to look at sort of in concert to see how we
can treat the cancer and also do it in a more specific way so
that the treatments are less and less toxic. I believe that if
the money is available for research, that these approaches
will be successful in the coming years...There's a lot of good
ideas out there and not everybody can get funding for those
ideas so those ideas go untested. You can't do the work
unless you have the money to do the research. The US is
falling behind other countries.

Paul Walker, M.D., Director of Oncology at the Brady School of
Medicine at East Carolina University expresses some concern about
the challenges ahead saying:

Now, from the treatment standpoint, it's sort of twofold.
Number one, is being able to better identify the genetic
makeup of an individual's cancer. That genetic makeup will
predict how it's going to behave, and then will ultimately provide the information on how to individualize the treatment...
The problem is that solid tumors are far more genomically
unstable - there is not going to be a magic pill for breast
cancer; there's not going to be a magic pill for lung cancer...Then we are talking about changing the survival time
of stage IV cancer from 10 months up to 30 months and
that in another itself is a gigantic advance. Just being able
to individualize and target personalized prognosis with

individualized treatment by targeting what's the problem in the first place...We have a lot of new therapies and there's a great rush in the pharmaceutical industry, all they want to do is get their drug approved as early as possible, and to be honest, there's a lot of cancer research that is geared toward advancing somebody's career, let's do something new because it seems to be pricey and sexy as opposed to we have a lot of other tools that haven't been properly used because there has been such a rush to focus on let's just target and see if we could find a magic bullet. We are not going to find a magic bullet for solid tumors.

Robert Bruno, Ph.D., Assistant Professor and Program Director of Molecular Diagnostics at Old Dominion University says:

There is a push now to get into more molecular analysis... Analyzing all the gene expressions of the cells in a biopsy which stratify patients into more complex groups...With the current standard of care, it's pretty limited in its use...the idea being, in the future, if we stratify patients that way at the molecular level you can better tailor treatment...really try to analyze the cells to see how the cancer is growing and functioning...I guess I am a little pessimistic...A lot of it is designing toxic chemotherapeutics, coming up with ways to target them to tumors...So it's not killing all the cells in your body but rather focusing on the tumor...Most molecularly targeted therapies have failed, in my opinion, largely because there is an incredibly amount of redundancy in a cell so if a cell is signaling through one pathway, we try to knock that down, it will try to find another way around it and that's kind of what happens. Tumors are incredibly heterogeneous and you take an average whenever you do an assessment of the tumors, you are looking at an average of all of the cells that you have selected but each cell is different so you might knock down one type of cell and another takes over.

There is some evidence that if you carefully alternate your chemotherapies to target [different types of cells] so you keep poking at different things that if you do it right it would turn it into a chronic illness rather than a deadly illness. I think one issue is that there is a little too much focus on the genetic aspect of the disease...and that's really been the focus of cancer research forever but I think what is being overlooked is the environmental influences on the cells and slowly but surely this is starting to gain steam with the bigger researchers who are pushing the idea that you need to start to look at it from a more holistic approach of targeting the cells that make up the environment around the tumors... You can reprogram tumor cells when you take them out of the tumor environment and put them in a different environment, a normal environment, you can get the cancer cells to start functioning normal which is really an incredible phenomenon. They have all the same mutations and everything but they're back to just behaving...Targeting is not a curative approach but rather turning it into a chronic illness...it can help in the short term but is not curative... I think there's too much attention to that and not enough to the broader basic questions in biology that we need to address and I think a lot of those can be addressed early on in terms of prevention of cancer.

Aliasger Salem, Ph.D., Professor of Pharmaceutical Science at the University of Iowa and Holden Comprehensive Cancer Center says:

Cancer immunotherapy basically uses the immune system to attack cancer cells that would otherwise be growing. It's sort of like, if you think about the flu or bacterial infection, your immune system could attack them to eliminate them. With the flu you can even vaccinate against the antigen so that the immune system is primed to get rid of that infection. The idea is that you could use the patient's own immune system to attack tumor cells that would progress into a solid cancer. This can be achieved through a couple of approaches. One of them is that you could immunize the patient directly using a vaccine...There are commercial products which treat the patient's immune system to recognize tumor cells as specific targets or you could use antibodies or adaptive T-cells to stimulate an immune response against that specific cancer. That is the basic idea. You are using the patient's own immune system to attack a specific cancer...It wouldn't have the same adverse side effects that chemotherapy would have because it is so targeted to a specific tumor that you are interested in. [Current] chemotherapy has an adverse effect on cancer cells but also an adverse effect on healthy cells so patients suffer these very, very serious side effects as part of the therapy such as hair loss, nausea, weakness, those types of things and they are pretty significant. With immunotherapy you would have reduced side effects relative to chemotherapy...An emerging area is adaptive T-cell therapy which is the idea of transfusing T-cells that have been trained to respond against the cancer and re-injecting them into patients to trigger an immune response against the cancer itself...In some cases, people have taken the T-cells from the patient and genetically engineered them and then put them back into the patient to respond against the cancer...There can be side effects and potential risks of immunotherapy such as immune disease, severe inflammatory response, fever...

Richard Heller, Ph.D., Professor of Medical Laboratory and Radiation Sciences at Old Dominion University says:

[In immunotherapy] we try to train the immune system to identify these cancer cells and then stimulate immune cells that go around the body looking for these cancer cells to destroy them. People have been chasing that for a long time... But that is really what we all strive for is to try to do that. Whether we will ever have complete success or not, I don't know. Right now the percentages are kind of low but what we hope for is to combine some of these agents and improve the approach to a point where it gets better and better...In immunotherapy, they take out the T-cells which are the immune cells that you want to stimulate and the ones that are already educated against the cancer. They can isolate those out and then sort of grow them in the laboratory and stimulate them and remove the rest of them from the person and then re-inject the T-cells back into the patient and these are primed and ready to go after any cancer cells and then they add other drugs that keep them stimulated. It is a very complex process... there is a lot of toxicity involved as well and the Holy Grail is to do it in such a way which is very easy for the patients and to get rid of it but of course that's easier said than done...We want to get to the point where we say we cured and I always hesitate to use that term because with cancer, it can come back, you can get it again.

Charlie Wei, Ph.D., Professor of Cellular and Molecular Biology and Immunology at Clemson University says:

Immunotherapy involves trying to engage a person's immune system to prevent and treat cancer. Early research is occurring to try to modulate the immune system to enhance activity... Research also demonstrates that people's natural immune system is already very involved in cancer prevention...In most cases, the immune system is able to see abnormal cells and eliminate them - that is what we call 'immune surveillance'...We believe immunotherapy will have less side effects than chemotherapy...That does not mean it will not have any side effects. In some situations we may face something like auto-immune problems. If your immune system is enhanced too much, it might start to target healthy tissues...It is still a young field of research and we have many unanswered questions which is why the FDA does not permit its use on early stage cancer patients.

Steven McMahon, Ph.D., Professor of Epigenetics at Thomas Jefferson University says:

The old-fashioned chemotherapy that just hits every rapidly dividing population of cells...is also going to get other systems in our bodies that have rapidly dividing cells...like our G.I. tract or our immune system...We will get away from just hitting every rapidly dividing cell with a sledgehammer and really just have this targeted effect on cancer...This gets a fast response but it's not durable...Cancer cells will figure out a way to get around the drug...So you get resistance to these drugs...so you need a second wave of different drugs which is a fixable problem...We have to do a lot more work I think...If multiple drugs can be given simultaneously to knock out secondary mutations, that might be considered a cure.

Ze'ev Ronai, Ph.D., Scientific Director of Sanford Burnham Laboratory says:

Prevention and delaying of metastasis is an area where I expect progress...This may have a major impact - keeping the cancer in check so metastasis does not occur...Today the likelihood of taking a drug to prevent cancer is very, very low but in the future based on the genetic analysis of the cancer, we will hopefully have the drugs to deal with those mutations. Prevention should not only be what we can do in our life to prevent cancer but also what we can do once cancer develops to prevent metastasis...That's where I foresee interventions being more effective...and prolonging your life...The degree of toxicity will be reduced substantially with targeted chemotherapy aimed at certain gene mutations based on genetic analysis using specific drugs designed for those mutations. Maybe 5 to 10 years from now we will be in a much better position. I want to emphasize I am not talking about a cure...Targeted chemotherapy will be used in conjunction with immunotherapy in the future...

Radiation Therapy

Similar to targeted chemotherapy and immunotherapy, the treatment of cancer by radiating tumors also strives to improve focus on the diseased tissue while protecting surrounding diseased tissue. Howard Gross, M.D., Medical Oncologist with the Dayton Clinical Oncology Program says, "In radiation therapy, they are always developing new techniques and are improving safety...". Nicole Simone, M.D., a Radiation Oncologist at Thomas Jefferson University says that for some cancers, "We are using a very pinpoint radiation therapy...that decreases some toxicity to healthy tissues...the outcomes for the patients are about the same but the toxicity can be much less [with fewer side effects]."

Treatment of Childhood Cancers

Some real and substantial progress has already been made with treatment of childhood cancers relative to the success of treatment of adult cancers. Gary Meadows, Ph.D., Professor of Pharmaceutical Science at Washington State University says, "We have had the most success curing cancers in children with chemotherapies and also some of the targeted therapies." Edward Trapido, Ph.D., Professor and Chair of Epidemiology at Louisiana School of Public Health explains:

The treatment for most childhood cancers is so great, terrific that deaths from childhood cancer have become much less common than they were. The main reason that's the case is because when a child has cancer and the doctor says there's a new medication out there that might help, 'Do you want to enroll your child?' The parent doesn't hesitate. Great progress has been made through clinical trials with children that have produced a large number of therapeutic agents and other ways of treating childhood cancers that have been very, very successful. That hasn't happened in adults. Adults are much less likely themselves to enroll in clinical trials and so the progress in treatment has not been nearly as great in adult cancers as they have been in childhood cancers.

Other Potential Future Developments

Will we be able to someday in the distant future be able to analyze people's genetic make-up and determine their cancer risks and make a plan of testing the patient specifically for those risks? East Carolina University's Paul Walker, M.D. hopes so saying:

If through some type of new technology, you knew you were at risk for lung cancer, you would get lung cancer screening, if you knew you were not at risk, you would not need that test...To be able to really identify who is at risk we could focus all of the resources even with the screening tools we have now...

John Bell, M.D., a surgical oncologist and Director of the Cancer Institute at the University of Tennessee hopes that in addition to today's important early detection techniques, that we can develop super-early cancer detection explaining:

I hope we reach a point where we can someday really advance molecular diagnostics and molecular therapeutics. In other words, finding disease at the microscopic or molecular level before it becomes detectable by current standards means...

and then hopefully be able to apply a therapy that would fix a gene that has gone awry or a metabolic pathway that has gone awry and get the patient back to a normal state of molecular health...That's where a lot of research is going these days...I really believe someday we will get there...I don't know that we will live to see it but I really believe our children will live to see the day where molecular diagnostics and therapeutics replace some of the more macro things we do today.

Another up and coming development to monitor in the coming years has to do with our relatively newfound knowledge pertaining to molecules called micro-RNAs (miRNAs). It is hoped that miRNA signatures will allow doctors to be able to target a treatment course. William Hendry, Ph.D., Professor and Chair of the Department of Biological Sciences at Wichita State University explains:

One other consideration to watch in the future is related to epigenetics. There is a whole new paradigm in science called non—coding RNA or micro-RNAs. I think there's a lot of evidence that they...will be used in diagnosis, prognosis as well as treatment of various types of diseases - particularly cancer in the future.

Perhaps in the future there will be ways to analyze people's genetic make-up for the purpose of telling them what environmental exposures to avoid. Stanford University's Alice Whittemore, Ph.D. says:

There certainly are examples where certain people with certain genetic factors have worse side effects from certain drugs and certain [environmental] exposures. I think we are going to learn a great deal more about that as time goes on with larger and larger studies and larger and larger sample sizes. We will find out, and I think this will be encouraging,

which people should avoid certain [environmental] exposures because of their genetic predispositions and which
other people can reasonably put that at the bottom of their
worry list, such and such an exposure. This is what our hope
is. Whether this is going to happen in the next 25 years, who
is to know.

11

Conclusion

What the brief section of this book on treatment tells us is that there are exciting, but uncertain, developments in cancer treatment that are being pursued throughout the country and throughout the world. As in any major technological endeavor, there are many technical hurdles that must yet be cleared if these treatments are to bear fruit and someday be able help millions of cancer patients worldwide. As we have heard from research experts above, some are optimistic while others have concerns or are outright pessimistic. For example, Carlos Sonnenschein, M.D., Professor of Integrative Physiology and Pathobiology at Tufts University School of Medicine says, "The cure for cancer has been promised every year for the last 40 years and the real cure doesn't have any reality. Therefore, why don't we convince our leaders to invest in prevention...". Some of the optimists have hope perhaps from recent advances in genomics, some successes in treating cancers in children and some successful targeted therapy with melanomas (skin cancer) noted in the treatment section of this book.

At a minimum, however, there is still a lot of uncertainty around cancer treatment advances and the likelihood is that, even if the technical hurdles are solved, we likely will have a number of years and possibly decades before they are successfully used on most cancer patients throughout the US and the rest of the world. Dale Shepard, M.D., Ph.D., a medical oncologist with the Cleveland Clinic explains of the new targeted treatments:

This will give us the ability to treat the right patient with the right drug...these developments will probably be in the 5 to 20 year range...It takes a while to get drugs through the approval process so that if they have not even yet gotten early phase drug trials that will easily be 5 to 7 years before they get tested in larger Phase 3 trials, get approved and really have some impact on patients...Immunotherapies are a little further along [than targeted chemotherapies]... There are some immunotherapies that have been approved for melanomas recently and really do offer some significant treatment options for patients - those are going to make an impact a lot faster.

It should be pointed out that a big question remains, even if these targeted treatments overcome many of the technical hurdles, will they only marginally improve life expectancy and quality of life or will the effects be much more dramatic with significant advances in those areas and maybe someday approximate a "cure" for cancer. Only time will tell.

In the meantime, 580,000 Americans are dying every year of cancer and over 8 million worldwide from what experts believe is a largely preventable disease - cancer. Since all cancer experts agree that it is better to not get cancer in the first place and given our increased knowledge about epigenetics, environmental causes of cancer and cancer prevention, it is incumbent upon all of us to do our part to use that knowledge to protect ourselves and our families. University of Kentucky's Susan Arnold, M.D. says, "We live in an era where the genomic understanding of human disease has exploded in the last 5 to 10 years, and that impacts environmental causes of cancer in ways that we never would have dreamed of in the 1950s so I think in that regard, it's more of a challenge but also more hope." University of North Carolina, Chapel Hill's Kurt Ribisl, Ph.D. adds, "People really do have the ability to substantially reduce their [cancer] risk".

However, just as there are hurdles in the arena of cancer treatment, so it is true of cancer prevention. One of those hurdles is that we need to remind our elected representatives that a healthy population is one of the foundations for a strong nation and we expect them to pursue public policy accordingly – whether it is policies that contribute to reduced tobacco use, overweight and obesity or cleaning up our environment. Carlos Crespo, Ph.D., Professor of Community Health at Portland State University says, "We made this environment and we can fix it again. We created what is killing us and we can fix it...".

Another challenge pertains to individual personal responsibility. That is, people have to do their best to take good care of themselves and their families. We have to educate a lot of people about what we know about cancer prevention and how to change their behaviors accordingly and as we all know, change is hard! The good news is that people are really interested in their health and many individuals and their families are starting to change. In fact, the number one use of search engines such as Google is researching topics on health. Many people do try to eat healthy and exercise. Each year Americans spend $1.5 billion on supplements and vitamins and the EPA says Americans spend billions on home water filtration units. The obesity epidemic in the US and some other countries is starting to level off. We have more people moving to largely plant-based diets with more vegetarians and vegans than ever before. Many supermarkets now have organic food sections reflecting the increased interest on the part of their customers. People would not be taking these steps if they did not care about their health.

This is at least a start but as this book has documented, many Americans are not doing as well with two-thirds being overweight or obese, millions being exposed to toxic environmental chemicals, still too many tobacco users, etc. While we have a long ways to go, people can improve themselves if they put their minds to it. It all starts with having an overall belief and philosophy in the importance of healthy living as an integral part of living a satisfying life. Plymouth State University's Barbara McCahan, Ph.D. explains:

> Eating a plant based diet, not eating too much, getting the physical activity you need, practicing safe sex, reducing your consumption of alcohol, not smoking - they are all linked together - a set of behaviors that comes from a value, a basic philosophy that works - it just works...It has a focus on a total set of values that changes your paradigm entirely.

Finally, just do the best you can – no reasonable person can ever ask more of you – and try to provide support and understanding to someone else close to you who may be struggling to make a positive change in his or her life but may be experiencing some setbacks as we all do from time to time. David LaPorte, Ph.D., Professor of Psychology at Indiana University of Pennsylvania points out that there is an expectation that if a person does not or cannot stop a detrimental health behavior, that there is something wrong with him or her and he or she is a failure adding:

> A spouse or family member can help buffer that, by saying, 'Look, I see that you are trying really hard and I know that it is difficult for you and no matter what happens, you are still a good person and I still love you, I still care for you.' Those kinds of things are important...

Most importantly, no matter what – love and respect yourself - you deserve it!

About the Author

Steve Riczo holds a Bachelor's Degree from Hiram College and Master's Degree in Healthcare Administration from Xavier University. He has 30 years of senior healthcare management experience, taught healthcare management at the University of Akron and is currently on the adjunct faculty of Cleveland State University and Kent State University. He is also a regular contributing author to *USA Today* magazine on healthcare issues and is the President and CEO of Riczo & Co., a healthcare consulting firm based in Cleveland, Ohio. Mr. Riczo may be contacted through the "Contact Us" page of his company web site at www.GlobalHealthOptions.net.

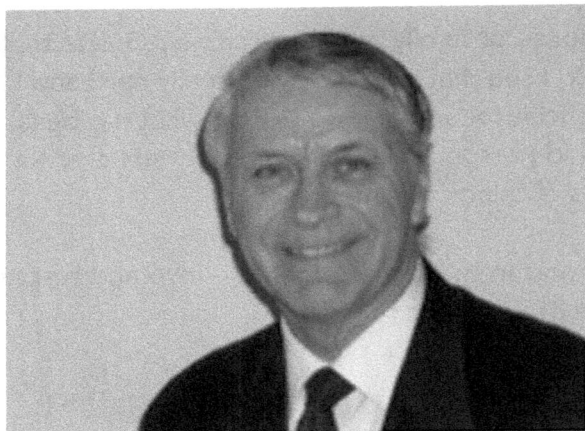

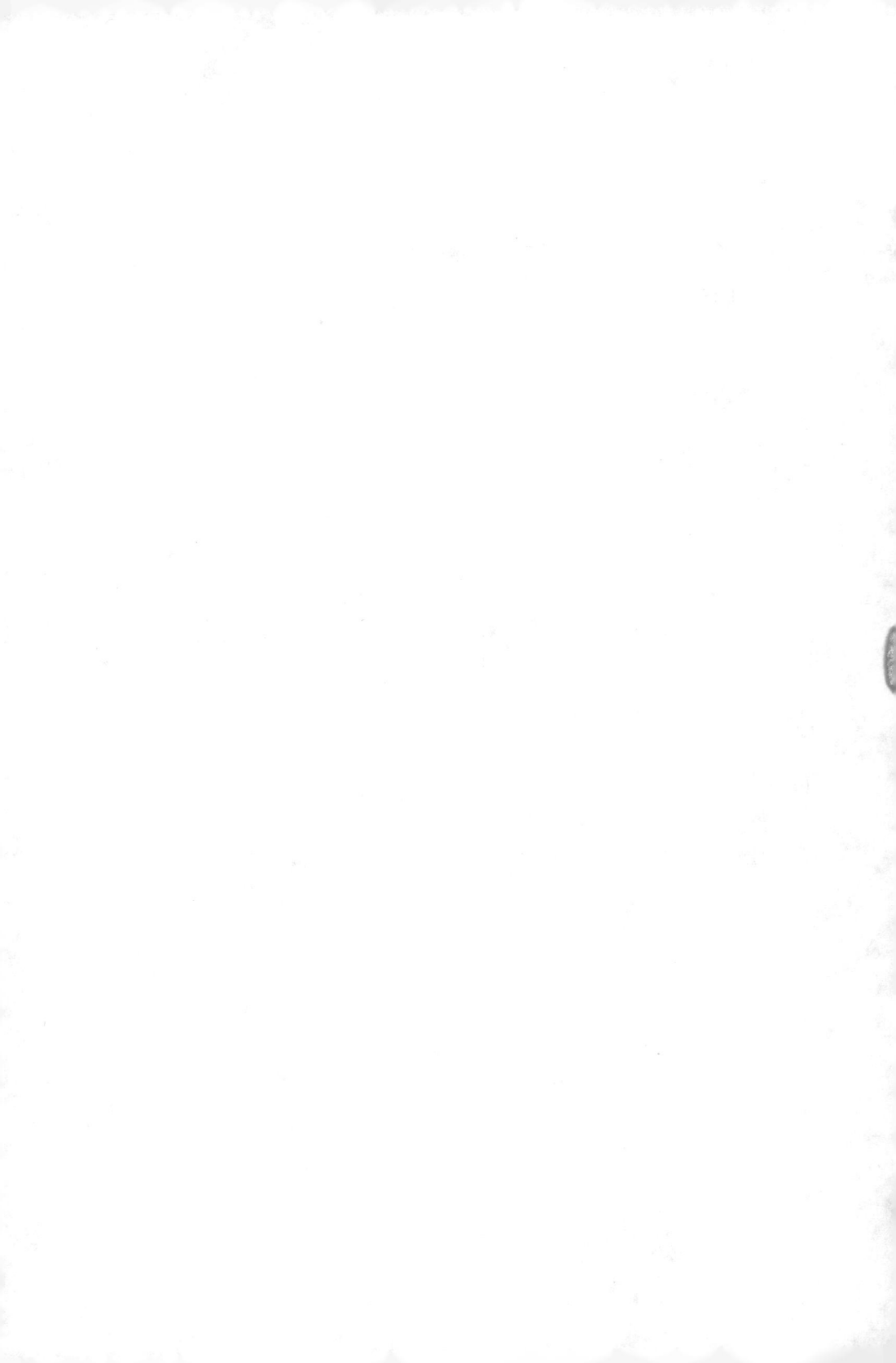

www.ingramcontent.com/pod-product-compliance
Lightning Source LLC
Chambersburg PA
CBHW072129270326
41931CB00010B/1717